Letters *from* Women in Pharmacy

Stories on Integrating Life and Career

EDITORS

Sara J. White, MS, FASHP
Director of Pharmacy (Ret.)
Stanford Hospital and Clinics
Past President, ASHP
Palo Alto, California
Faculty, ASHP Education and Research Foundation's
    Pharmacy Leadership Academy

Susan Teil Boyer, MS, FASHP
Senior Consultant, ASHP Consulting
Past Board Member, ASHP
Tacoma, Washington
Faculty, ASHP Education and Research Foundation's
    Pharmacy Leadership Academy

Hannah K. Vanderpool, PharmD, MA
Vice President, Office of Member Relations
ASHP
Bethesda, Maryland

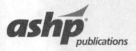

Any correspondence regarding this publication should be sent to the publisher, American Society of Health-System Pharmacists, 4500 East-West Highway, Bethesda, MD 20814, attention: Special Publishing.

The information presented herein reflects the opinions of the contributors and advisors. It should not be interpreted as an official policy of ASHP or as an endorsement of any product.

Because of ongoing research and improvements in technology, the information and its applications contained in this text are constantly evolving and are subject to the professional judgment and interpretation of the practitioner due to the uniqueness of a clinical situation. The editors and ASHP have made reasonable efforts to ensure the accuracy and appropriateness of the information presented in this document. However, any user of this information is advised that the editors and ASHP are not responsible for the continued currency of the information, for any errors or omissions, and/or for any consequences arising from the use of the information in the document in any and all practice settings. Any reader of this document is cautioned that ASHP makes no representation, guarantee, or warranty, express or implied, as to the accuracy and appropriateness of the information contained in this document and specifically disclaims any liability to any party for the accuracy and/or completeness of the material or for any damages arising out of the use or non-use of any of the information contained in this document.

Acquisitions Editor: Daniel Cobaugh

Editorial Project Manager, Special Publishing: Ruth Bloom

Production Manager: Johnna Hershey

Cover & Page Design: David Wade

Library of Congress Cataloging - in - Publication Data

Names: White, Sara J., 1945- editor. | Boyer, Susan Teil, editor. | Vanderpool, Hannah K., editor. | American Society of Health-System Pharmacists.
Title: Letters from women in pharmacy: stories on integrating life and career / editors, Sara J. White, Susan Teil Boyer, Hannah K. Vanderpool.
Description: Bethesda, MD : American Society of Health-System Pharmacists, [2019]
Identifiers: LCCN 2018034779 | ISBN 9781585286126 (pbk.)
Subjects: | MESH: Pharmacy | Women | Collected Correspondence
Classification: LCC RM301.15 | NLM WZ 112.5.P4 | DDC 615.1--dc23
LC record available at https://lccn.loc.gov/2018034779

Printed in Canada.

ISBN: 978-1-58528-612-6

10 9 8 7 6 5 4 3 2 1

Dedication

To the courageous women who want it all:

We challenge you to always push societal and personal boundaries to define a woman's place on your own terms.

Dear Shannan,　　　July 31, 2020

I am grateful to have been your RPD and now colleague & friend.

Many wonderful adventures lie before you personally and professionally.

Many Blessings!

Patti

Acknowledgments

We want to express our sincere appreciation to Daniel Cobaugh, Ruth Bloom, Johnna Hershey, and their colleagues in ASHP's Publishing Division for their guidance and patience throughout the development and production of this book.

Thank you for the generosity of these women who shared their personal and professional vulnerabilities and passions in these letters to benefit current and future leaders in pharmacy.

A Note from the Editors

The vision for this book is to support successful women leaders through the power of personal stories. By creating an awareness of the daily struggles and resilience of a cross-section of ASHP member leaders, current and future generations of women may identify themselves in these stories and find encouragement for their own leadership journey.

Contents

Preface

The ASHP 2016 Women in Pharmacy Leadership Steering Committee's recommendation to ASHP to *"proactively collect and share stories, case studies and scenarios of how women have addressed gender, workplace, work–life integration, and leadership challenges"* was the impetus and stimulus for this *Letters* publication. The power of this publication comes from each letter writer's personal journey, each unique yet similar, in reaching for her potential as both a pharmacist and as a woman. The letters collectively emphasize the numerous successful approaches to blending a career and personal life while learning and applying various leadership styles.

We (Sara, Susan, and Hannah) as co-editors sought out women pharmacists who bring out a multiplicity of voices in age, cultural and ethnic backgrounds, practice settings, and work and personal experiences. A strong common theme heard by the Steering Committee was the need to learn more about integration of career and life. We sought women who represented a variety of personal life circumstances, such as single/married, with and without children, divorced, single mom, stay-at-home dad, and diverse lifestyles to cast a wide net to benefit our readers.

With our colleagues, co-workers, and friends, we too often focus on portraying our successes, while minimizing or hiding our fears, challenges, failures, or pain. As life happens, you will find journeys that include health challenges, job layoffs, changing jobs, overcoming humble beginnings, going back to school, and benefiting from the resilience of others, such as having a mother who survived the Auschwitz WWII concentration camp. We asked these contributors to share advice on overcoming gender-limiting and societal assumptions, self-doubt, guilt, imposter syndrome, rejection, failures, and #MeToo moments. You will find how the value of saying both "yes" and "no," the decision to risk change, the value of seizing opportunities, and letting go of the pharmacist perfectionist in the other aspects of life are beneficial. These letter writers also share how mentors, networking, volunteering in professional organizations, and investment of time and attention into relationships outside of their friends and family have positively shaped their lives and careers.

This *Letters from Women in Pharmacy: Stories on Integrating Life and Career* joins ASHP's other books of letters: *Letters to a Young Pharmacist: Sage Advice on Life & Career from Extraordinary Pharmacists* (mid-career to veterans) (Susan A. Cantrell, Sara J. White, and Bruce E. Scott), *Letters from Rising Pharmacy*

Stars: Advice on Creating and Advancing Your Career in a Changing Profession (10+ years of practice) (Susan A. Cantrell and Sara J. White), and *Letters from Pharmacy Residents: Navigating Your Career* (Sara J. White, Harold N. Godwin, and Susan Teil Boyer). These books were the brainchild of Susan Cantrell who had read Ellyn Spragins' books that featured authors writing letters to their younger selves. Susan talked to Sara about using the concept for pharmacy, which has resulted in this family of letters books.

We hope these stories, journeys, and practical advice will help you realize that others support and understand the challenges of your journey as you push through any guilt, self-doubt, and the inevitable obstacles to having a satisfying career and personal life.

Enjoy,

Sara, Susan, and Hannah

Introduction

Imperative for Change

The Pharmacy Workforce Center commissioned the 2014 National Pharmacist Workforce Study that revealed, for the first time in history, pharmacy shifted from a male-dominated to a female-dominated profession.[1] In addition, over the last 20 years, pharmacy school enrollment of women has increased, representing 62.5% of all first professional degree students, and 52.6% of all full-time graduate pharmacy students.[2] With women graduating from pharmacy school at higher rates and men retiring at a much faster rate than women, it became more apparent that ASHP should study the potential implications of this shift.

Although the data show that women represent the majority of healthcare practitioners today, they still occupy far fewer leadership positions in healthcare at large, particularly at senior leadership levels. A separate study on women and leadership, conducted by the Pew Research Center, found that key leadership traits such as intelligence and capacity for innovation are indistinguishable from men and women.[3]

ASHP Women in Pharmacy Leadership Initiative

ASHP sought to respond to the evolving environment to anticipate the needs and changing dynamics of the pharmacy workforce. In 2015, the Women in Pharmacy Leadership Initiative was launched with the Women in Pharmacy Leadership Steering Committee. The Committee members (both women and men) represented a diverse group of pharmacy leaders from a variety of practice settings and positions in a wide range of career stages. They were charged with exploring possible recommendations to support women in achieving pharmacy leadership skills and roles at every level and practice setting. Through various means, such as empirical studies, focus groups, town hall meetings, and open discussion sessions, the Committee formed a set of recommendations focused on leveraging the change in demographics as a business and leadership opportunity for the profession.

The ASHP Board of Directors in 2016 approved the Steering Committee report, which contained the following series of recommendations.

Recommendations to ASHP:

1. Allocate resources strategically to create and sustain specific ASHP services including meetings and education, skills building programs, networking forums to support career development strategies, and other resources.

2. Identify and share strategies for successful work–life integration with members. Work–life integration is an ongoing issue for all pharmacy professionals (men and women).

3. Highlight the differences between role models, mentors, coaches, and sponsors and foster the development of these relationships among its members. Specifically, the concept of sponsorship should be introduced and nurtured between early female careerists and successful women leaders.

4. Develop a strategy to collect baseline and ongoing metrics regarding women in leadership positions within the pharmacy profession. Data exist within the general workforce and within healthcare but not within the pharmacy profession.

5. Proactively collect and share stories, case studies, and scenarios of how women have addressed gender, workplace, work–life integration, and leadership challenges.

6. Assess volunteer, meeting, and governance policies and practices to support successful engagement and participation among ASHP members.

7. Share successful pharmacy employer policies and practices that reflect supportive work environments.

8. Study pharmacy-specific career inflection points including individual, organizational, and societal factors and promote these leverage points.

9. Cultivate career aspirations of early careerists.

10. Facilitate leadership development throughout all functional roles (e.g., clinical, administrative, academic).

11. Actively recruit women into its elected and appointed leadership and support their advancements by recognizing their volunteer contributions and achievements.

12. Support ASHP state affiliates and colleges of pharmacy in disseminating and supporting the Women in Pharmacy Leadership recommendations at the school, local, and state level.

Recommendations to Those Seeking Leadership Roles:

1. Develop a strategic career plan focused on personal skill development, and meet with senior leaders to voice aspirations.
2. Seek applicable education and training (e.g., advanced degrees, residency training, skills-based leadership training) to support career trajectory.
3. Recognize that one's career progression is a journey and that each transition entails a new level of commitment and dedication to work–life integration.
4. Expand a network of seasoned practitioners both male and female.
5. Identify mentors and sponsors and nurture productive relationships.
6. Be assertive in negotiating, designing, and applying work models that meet the needs of employers as well as individual professional and personal needs for work–life balance.

Recommendations to Current Pharmacy Leaders:

1. For individuals who are in the position of mentoring and sponsoring others, actively identify mentees and nurture those who would benefit from sponsorship, working together to create a personal development plan.
2. Promote key factors that create positive career changes such as advanced degrees and residency training (career inflection points) among mentees.
3. Encourage aspiring leaders to seek and take on visible, important, and complex roles and projects.
4. Make introductions of aspiring leaders with other influential leaders.
5. Provide specialized coaching and give feedback.
6. Support the expansion of professional networks of emerging leaders.
7. Share profiles, stories, and recommendations of successful female pharmacy leaders with others.

Recommendations to Employer Organizations/Pharmacy Departments:

1. Cultivate career aspirations of female early careerists.
2. Encourage early careerists to proactively manage career plans.
3. Develop mentoring, coaching, and sponsorship programs.
4. Promote active assumption of sponsorship activities to advance aspiring leaders.
5. Identify challenges that prevent aspiring women leaders from pursuing advanced career goals.

6. Create and expand residency programs and other skills-based formal educa-tion and training programs, including leadership training, that have been shown to be instrumental in career success.

7. Examine and consider implementation of organizational policies to provide support to working professionals including flexible hours, job sharing, etc.

8. Offer and/or support education, training programs, and personal develop-ment opportunities to build success skills.

The work of the Committee and subsequent recommendations became the cata-lyst for other activities in support of the Women in Pharmacy Leadership Initia-tive. A variety of communication channels and facilitation methods have since been used to establish ongoing services and member engagement. Networking sessions at ASHP national meetings connect those interested in the Initiative and facilitate mentorship/sponsorship, and educational sessions on leadership topics keep members apprised of the unique needs of women and those in lead-ership positions.

To communicate the progress of the Initiative and to serve as a home for those seeking to learn more and engage in the conversation, the following were created:

- A web page (https://www.ashp.org/Pharmacy-Practice/Resource-Centers/Leadership/Women-In-Pharmacy-Leadership)
- A dedicated online discussion forum—the ASHP Connect Women in Phar-macy Leadership Community

Information sharing has also increased to continue to raise awareness and promote member activities through:

- Podcasts
- Newsletters such as Intersections (http://www.ashpintersections.org/)
- Social media

In continuing ASHP's tradition of learning and inspiration through engage-ment and education, a commentary on Women in Pharmacy Leadership was commissioned for the *American Journal of Health-System Pharmacy* to contribute to the body of knowledge on the topic.

This broad and in-depth engagement strategy to stimulate courageous conversations about gender diversity and leadership needs was highly successful for ASHP. Utilizing a variety of communication channels and facilitation methods yielded strong consensus around the needs of current and future leaders of the profession. New programs created during this initiative have been established as ongoing services, and the uptake of these services by ASHP members have been significant. This initiative contributes to ASHP's goal to support and encourage our members through their personal and professional leadership journeys.

Maria Carias and Hannah K. Vanderpool

References

1. National Pharmacist Workforce Study. April 8, 2015. https://www.aacp.org/sites/default/files/finalreportofthenationalpharmacistworkforcestudy2014.pdf. Accessed October 9, 2018.

2. American Association of Colleges of Pharmacy. Academic Pharmacy's Vital Statistics. July 2018. https://www.aacp.org/article/academic-pharmacys-vital-statistics. Accessed October 9, 2018.

3. Pew Research Center, Social & Demographic Trends. Women and Leadership: Public Says Women Are Equally Qualified, but Barriers Persist. January 14, 2015. http://www.pewsocialtrends.org/2015/01/14/women-and-leadership/. Accessed October 9, 2018.

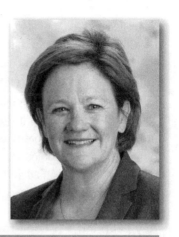

Tina Aramaki
PharmD, MBA

Plan Your Career Course, but Be Open to Unexpected Paths

Tina is an experienced pharmacy leader who shares her insights and experiences from her professional journey during her years in health-system pharmacy. She currently serves as Vice President of Banner Health's Pharmacy Division. Tina also served on the Board of Trustees for Roseman University of the Health Sciences, Jordan, Utah and Henderson, Nevada.

Tina holds a BS degree in Pharmacy (1980) from the University of Utah, a PharmD (2002) from the University of Florida, and an MBA from North Central University in Phoenix, Arizona.

Tina's advice is: Look for potential in others. There is always something to learn. Don't allow comfort to get in the way of opportunity. Be open to new adventures.

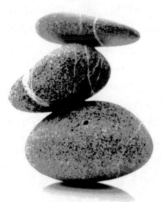

Dear Colleague,

I'm excited to share experiences from my journey as a pharmacist and pharmacy leader. I couldn't have anticipated or planned the course I have taken, so if there is an overarching theme for this letter, it would be to plan your course but be open to unexpected paths that will lead to your destination!

Beginning my career, I was excited to work in a staff/clinical role in a small community hospital.

1

My colleagues and I developed our practice in ways that were quite advanced for the time, particularly in that setting. We had developed pharmacy and therapeutics (P&T) approved protocols that allowed our clinical pharmacists to manage all total parenteral nutrition (TPN), aminoglycoside and vancomycin dosing, as well as collaborating with physicians on antimicrobial stewardship. I was eager to continue my career as a hospital pharmacist and develop my relationship with/ provide service to my patients as well as nursing and physician colleagues. Traditional shiftwork enabled me to work part-time hours when I was raising small children. I hadn't considered a career path in management or even seen myself as a formal leader. I was very content with my career.

Key Learning #1: Look for potential in others, and help them identify opportunities they might not otherwise recognize.

During a regular one-on-one visit, my pharmacy leader pointed out that I had become an informal leader of the staff. The department relied on me professionally for setting a tone and culture of quality improvement, safety, and positivity. I developed great relationships with our medical and nursing staffs. The pharmacy director pointed out that this made me a leader, and he encouraged me to consider additional leadership roles. When an opportunity presented itself, I was encouraged to apply for the position of Director of Pharmacy. The hospital administrator also reached out to me with a similar encouraging message. He believed I would be the leader they needed. Although my children were in school full days, I was a bit nervous about going back to work full time. My husband and I discussed how my career change might impact our family, and we made a joint decision that I should apply. During the interview process, I felt like I was getting cold feet. I wasn't certain that what I had to offer was enough. I had that discussion with my former leader, and he encouraged me to continue on my path.

As I was selected for the role and began developing our department and staff, I became more self-confident. In my career up to this point, these were leaders I respected who identified strengths that I wouldn't have recognized in myself. Through their vision, I was able to grow and develop. I became a positive influence as a mentor; I have consistently sought to help my colleagues, employees, students, and residents identify their strengths and skills and to seek opportunities that may seem beyond their reach. People don't always recognize their potential, and it is important for others to help them both appreciate and achieve that potential.

Key Learning #2: Don't allow comfort to get in the way of opportunity.

I was happy in the Director of Pharmacy role. I was growing as a leader and as a pharmacist, and my job felt like home. In an informal role, I had proactively brought together the pharmacy directors from my multihospital health system in our geographic region to collaborate on issues of policy and clinical pharmacy standards. In our meetings, each of the directors had a lot to contribute. We were finding opportunities for improvement throughout the healthcare system. It occurred to me that there were opportunities for leadership beyond those of leading one hospital pharmacy.

At this time, I made the decision to continue my formal education by completing a nontraditional PharmD degree. Our two sons were in middle and high school, so I also hoped to be a good example of discipline in studying and academic achievement. The boys were NOT impressed, but I succeeded in completing my advanced degree. As a woman and mother, I have often sought greater meaning or benefit from my own endeavors. In furthering my education, I moved out of my comfort zone and hopefully impacted my children and their thirst for learning.

As I thought about my future, I really believed I would continue working as Director of Pharmacy at the same hospital. But a great friend of mine pointed out that if I wanted to move to that next level of leadership, I would probably have to move to Tennessee, headquarters for HCA Healthcare. He then suggested I look at a similarly-sized hospital searching for a pharmacy director within Intermountain Healthcare. Because the headquarters was in Salt Lake City, where I lived, there was more opportunity for advancement. It was a tough decision to make, as I had spent 20 years building my practice and relationships. I had to decide about trading comfort for opportunity. My friend was right. After working in the Intermountain Healthcare Community Hospital for two years, I received a promotion to a system manager role, and then to the System Director of Pharmacy for Intermountain Healthcare.

Key Learning #3: If you want to impact your patients and other pharmacists and technicians, become a leader. If you want to impact generations of patients and pharmacists, become a residency leader. And this key learning is a "two-fer." Understand that whatever you teach others, you will get back in multiples.

At Intermountain, I was learning so much and developing relationships with my colleagues and a whole new set of skills. I learned an integrated approach to policy, clinical practices, and care of patients. The practices and learnings became a passion. We were finding new efficiency and effectiveness in sharing skills and expertise between hospitals and clinicians, as well as creating consistency in care across the continuum of patients' lives. I believed I had reached the pinnacle of my career. A close friend and colleague (yes, this is becoming a trend!) challenged me to develop a postgraduate year 1 and 2 (PGY 1 and 2) health-system pharmacy administration residency. I really doubted my capabilities to lead a residency, as I had never completed a residency myself. But with the help and guidance of my colleague, and with the support of my residents, *we* developed the residency. I began working toward sharing the knowledge and experience I had gained over the prior 27 years with our residents. What a great opportunity! We created consistent training programs for technicians and inventory management solutions for hospitals. We developed a deep appreciation for providing service excellence that impacted the acceptance of ambulatory clinical services. The experiences I gained during the ensuing seven years, and seven resident graduates, provided fulfillment beyond my dreams. Our residency program was paired with an advanced leadership degree, so I was again inspired to seek *another* advanced degree that helped to develop my leadership capabilities. Imagine setting out to mentor pharmacy professionals and having them mentor you right back! I learned invaluable lessons from these amazing professionals, and some of them continue mentoring me.

Key Learning #4: Be creative in achieving your dreams, while keeping a sharp eye on what is most important. If what you do professionally doesn't bring you closer to those you love, then do something else!

If I had finished my career at Intermountain Healthcare, I would have been very satisfied with my journey. But again, a colleague reached out to me saying Banner Health in Phoenix, Arizona, was looking for a Vice President of Pharmacy Services. Banner was looking for a pharmacy leader to develop an integrated pharmacy division. If I was selected, I would use everything I had learned from more than 30 years in practice to move another organization to new levels of success. I would also have the opportunity to establish a new health-system pharmacy administration residency program to become, again, a residency leader.

As I mentioned earlier, I really didn't want to relocate. I loved where I lived, and all of my family was there. My husband, also a pharmacist, was nearing the end of a successful career of his own. We couldn't move ... could we?

The decision we made is not one that would work for everyone. We knew that many people travel for work and are on the road Monday through Friday every week. When I accepted the position at Banner, we kept our home in Salt Lake City and bought a small condominium in Phoenix, very close to my office. I jokingly tell my colleagues that even with the 90-minute flight to and from Phoenix weekly, my total commute time is shorter than many! Thanks to technology, vacations, and occasionally working remotely, my husband and I are enjoying this adventure.

I don't know how much longer I will continue in my role at Banner Health, but just like my experience with establishing the residency program, I have gained much more than I have given. I have developed a more disciplined approach to leadership and accountability, but learned to maintain emotional connection with those I lead. I am focused on helping others achieve their potential and am again working as part of our health-system pharmacy administration residency to develop tomorrow's leaders. I have learned to surround myself with professionals who make me better, accentuate my strengths, and help mitigate my weaknesses.

I hope some of what I have learned will benefit you in your career.

Remember,

- Be curious and brave.

- Learn and teach.

- Be disciplined and creative.

- Be open to *new* adventures, while clinging to those that bring you strength and joy!

Kindest regards,

Tina

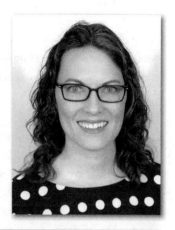

Jennifer (Jenny) Arnold
PharmD, BCPS

Are You Going Places or Being Taken?

Jenny is a pharmacist who is definitely going places. In her letter, Jenny describes the compelling path to her current role as Director of Practice Development, Washington State Pharmacy Association.

Jenny received her BS in Microbiology at the University of Washington and her PharmD degree (2006) also at the University of Washington, School of Pharmacy. Jenny completed an ASHP-accredited pharmacy residency at Swedish Medical Center, Seattle, Washington.

Jenny's advice is: I hope you are going places and not being taken. Find your passion and live it. Walk down your path with the confidence and grace that you have worked so hard to achieve.

Dear Colleague,

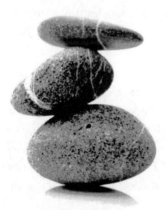

Are you going places or being taken? This statement was on a daily inspiration desk calendar that I read at just the right time in my life. I felt like I was waiting to be taken, and I was fed up by it. That simple quote led me to find the profession of pharmacy, my wonderful husband, and an internal strength and drive guiding me to this day. *How could one quote do all those things?* At that time, I wanted to climb and be surrounded by rocks and mountains in the Pacific Northwest, so I decided to take a climbing class. During a climb up Guye

Peak, Lynda Tanagi, a pharmacist at the University of Washington Medical Center, told me about her profession, and I have never looked back. One of my good friends took the climbing class with me, and he is now my husband. That climbing class helped me reach many summits in my life!

During pharmacy school I intended to be an inpatient pharmacist, most likely in the intensive care unit (ICU). I enjoyed working with the ICU's health-care team and solving unique pharmacologic challenges in acutely ill patients. I had a wonderful internship in a small hospital with strong mentors who are now friends. I completed a residency at a larger health system, but in the spring during my residency year, I was spun around completely on my axis. In the ICU I saw the same patients return with chronic obstructive pulmonary disease and chronic heart failure exacerbation who wouldn't be there if they had access to the right medications and education. This was before reducing readmission or transitions of care efforts. I realized that I needed to leave the inpatient setting so I could work to keep people *out* of the hospital. I transitioned to a unique role in an independent community pharmacy. There, I could use my clinical knowledge to help patients in their homes understand and take their medications—and I know I kept them out of the hospital. I was also able to establish new collaborative practice protocols, expand our vaccine recommendations, and more.

Moving to the community was scary for me. Although I had many amazing community pharmacist mentors, I had never pictured myself as one. I soon realized and respected the breadth of knowledge a community pharmacist has; they must know almost all the medications! No longer did I have the luxury of having a tremendous depth of knowledge about relatively few medications and guidelines. I had to know medications differently, thinking about patient counseling points and long-term side effects. However, the system I had developed during my residency to learn and use resources prepared me for this change. My experience in the inpatient setting was essential for helping patients transition after hospitalization and troubleshoot medication discrepancies. I was able to leverage partnerships with medical practitioners I met on the inpatient side into initiatives for the community setting.

Another unplanned opportunity presented itself a few years later. I was asked to apply for the Director of Practice Development position at the Washington State Pharmacy Association (WSPA). I had been an active member in the association since I was a student. Working for the WSPA would allow me to help Washington state pharmacists innovate and create new clinical roles. I was highly motivated to explore how pharmacists could bill for patient care, such as the care I had provided through the community pharmacy, and I was excited by the prospect of giving back to the association that had built so many bridges for me in my early career.

Working for the WSPA has taught me the power of advocacy. It also taught me how relationships you establish may come back to provide opportunities months or even years later. I follow legislation that I am passionate about, and I do not hesitate to reach out to my state or national representative with positive or negative feedback about a topic. I have testified on bills at the state level that I want to support or oppose and am very thankful to our CEO and our Director of Government Affairs for holding my hand the first few times I did it. My work has also made me appreciate the importance of the rules process. Our State Boards of Pharmacy need our input to make rules that protect patients and allow our profession to innovate to improve patient care. My role in crafting and advocating for rules and legislation, including ESSB 5557 passed in 2015 requiring insurance plans to add pharmacists as medical providers, has truly made me feel empowered. This legislation has opened a new path for the profession in our state.

Pharmacists are often intimidated by advocacy, but here are a few ideas to get started:

- *First, stay informed.* Find news sources and updates that help inform you as a voter, citizen, and professional. A free press is key to a strong democracy!

- *Second, attend your State Board of Pharmacy meetings.* Please stand up when they need clarification you can offer, or you have an idea to improve what they are working on. Ask people around you questions about the process so you feel comfortable there. Whether you are a director of pharmacy or a new graduate working as a staff pharmacist, your Board of Pharmacy needs you. If you cannot attend Board meetings, send in your feedback on their rules in process; they will use it.

- *Third, join.* Be a member of your local, state, and national or alumni association. Read their publications and attend a meeting periodically to connect with your peers. Your association values your support, and you will be better for the networking and connection to your profession. I am biased, as well as an extrovert and natural joiner, but my association engagement has given me endless opportunities and gratification.

- *Fourth, follow the legislation you care about.* Subscribe to the legislative updates from your association or legislator. If you care about a proposed bill, write a letter or set a meeting to share your thoughts with your council member, representative, or senator. Your association can share speaking points if needed.

My job includes boundless opportunities and projects with no true endpoint. Although I love my work, I am not a workaholic, and there is always a tug of war between my personal and professional life. The phrase "work–life balance" never made sense to me. I imagined a two-sided scale with the hours of a long day I just worked on one side and an equal number of hours at home on the other side. But sometimes there are not that many hours in a day. Instead, my wise aunt Pam said she strove for *sustainability*. She told me when work needed to be the priority, put my energy there. She also said, "I know you always give 120%, and when you need to pull back from work to recharge your batteries, feel good about doing that." I continue to follow this advice, more often now that I am a mom. After working long days, weekends, or traveling for work, I know that it is OK to leave work early for a day to run errands, attend the preschool party, or sleep. I know that I earned it, and it makes what I do sustainable. It avoids burnout. I employ this strategy at the WSPA where I am always looking for continuing education speakers and members to participate or lead meetings and work groups. When someone tells me they are spread too thin and cannot help, I say thank you and remind them our profession will always need leaders so to just let me know when they are ready. I think this helps to recharge them; they, too, must lead the path of their own life.

Being a slightly older parent has given me the privilege of watching the successes and challenges of my friends as parents. I realized how fast kids grow and change, and to appreciate each moment from them. What I did not realize as a working parent was how much I would miss the occasional late evenings spent cranking on a project. Now I need to be home for dinner and bedtime. Dinner is followed by washing the dishes, cleaning the house, and talking about the day with my husband Mike. The idea of working for a mere 30 minutes before bedtime is just not worth the effort to get out the computer and log on. Therefore, to compensate, I have become more productive *during* the work day by making better use of my time and being more particular about the tasks I take on.

I am typical among my female colleagues in that most of us must balance a two-career household. When your spouse not only works outside the home but also is building his own career, communication and compromises over schedules and priorities are a weekly and yearly discussion. Mike (who is not a pharmacist) has a job that, like mine, has periodic early mornings, late evenings, and travel. We send each other calendar reminders to coordinate schedules. The more understanding I am of his schedule, the more he reflects this back to me and my needs. We also call on our "village," which includes our nanny and many family members, to make it work. To say Mike and I are naturally chatty is an understatement, and we channel this into talking each evening about our day, our challenges, and our wins. We feed off each other's excitement and experiences. We make sure that we are on the same path.

So, colleague, I hope you lead your own path. I hope you are going places and not being taken. Find your passion and live it. Identify the gaps in your knowledge or practice and fix it. I hope you advocate for yourself and our profession. Surround yourself with family, friends, and colleagues who nurture and support you. Remember to walk down your path with the confidence and grace that you have worked so hard to achieve.

Take care,

Jenny

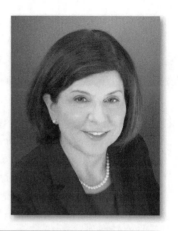

Katherine Benderev
PharmD, MBA

Work Successfully through Your Challenging Life Decisions

Kathy's career as a pharmacy professional and entrepreneur spans more than 25 years in management, administrative, consulting, and academic positions. She is currently a Senior Consultant to ASHP. In her letter, Kathy shares her insight on tackling life's toughest challenges.

Kathy earned her PharmD (1979) from the University of Maryland School of Pharmacy in Baltimore and her MBA from the University of California, Irvine. Kathy completed a residency in pharmacy practice at the University of California, San Diego, and a second-year residency in health-system pharmacy administration at Long Beach Memorial Medical Center in Long Beach, California.

Kathy's advice is: No matter how big the challenge, I can find a way forward by working through fears and doubts that potentially keep me stuck. Using a five-step fear-processing technique will help you to tackle and resolve difficult professional and personal decisions.

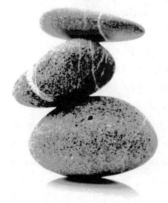

Dear Colleague,

I have been a hospital pharmacy manager throughout most of my career. I also taught pharmacy administration topics at the college level to both PharmD and Master's students. Consulting in health-system pharmacy and with medical device start-up companies has added to my work in healthcare. You could say I have truly taken advantage of opportunities the profession of pharmacy provides.

In this letter, I will share key milestones from my professional and personal life that became opportunities for growth and lessons learned. Techniques I have used to take advantage of new undertakings may help you, too.

How does someone identify when opportunities come their way? They may not be perceived as opportunities at the time. If you are so busy and lack time to reflect, opportunities will likely pass you by. Opportunities occur when you are actively thinking and open to new experiences. Capturing an opportunity may mean saying yes to an offer or making a choice that makes you feel uncomfortable. If the uncomfortable feeling involves true lack of interest, then it is usually best to move on. If the uncomfortable feeling has fear-related components to it, but some interest, then please continue reading as I might have a technique to help you deal with your fear and seize the opportunity. I discovered that being open to opportunities and actually learning the lessons means you have to deal with and work through fears and doubts rather than push them aside.

What were examples of my opportunities for growth and learning, and what were some fears and doubts I had to process? I began to develop my technique for dealing with fears early on as a student and then resident. One opportunity came when I was a pharmacy student at the University of Maryland as I considered applying for the recently introduced PharmD program. A few other states offered a PharmD degree, but *would there be jobs? How far would I have to move to get a job? How would I pay for graduate school?* I did not think I would succeed. But after receiving encouragement from one professor and choosing to step out of my comfort zone, I applied and was accepted into the third class of the University's PharmD program.

While in the PharmD program, I was faced with the decision of applying for a residency at the same time I was about to marry a medical student. Fears of leaving my home town, the anxiety of performing up to the standards of a post-graduate year 1 (PGY1) residency, and having a good marriage all at the same time were overwhelming. I wrote out all of my options with pros and cons for each and decided to apply for the residency and was accepted. Emboldened with the successes of being accepted into a competitive graduate program and residency and encouraged by my mentors, I applied for a PGY2 pharmacy administrative residency. I really wanted this opportunity, but I had to work through my fears of not being good enough. Again, I wrote down my concerns and consequences of action or inaction, applied, and was accepted. By being vulnerable and facing possible failure, I had actually accomplished my goals.

How did I work through all the decisions when I had a fear of failure, doubt about my skills, and knowledge and performance anxiety? At that time, I began to develop a method that I recently discovered is very similar to Tim Ferriss's "Fear-Setting" technique. (If you want more information on this technique, see his TED talk and don't let the beginning of the talk scare you: **https://www.ted. com/talks/tim_ferriss_why_you_should_define_your_fears_instead_of_ your_goals.**)

What I learned to do with my fears and doubts involved a five-step process that I call *fear-processing*. **The first step**: Write down my fears. I was very specific. For example, when I applied to the PGY2 residency, I wrote "I have a fear of being embarrassed in front of my peers and colleagues if I don't get accepted." Another fear was "What if I am accepted and I do a poor job, disappoint my preceptors, and ruin my reputation?"

The second step: Write down what I could do to prevent the likelihood of each fear materializing. I identified that no one had ever died from embarrassment and that failure was a way to learn and improve myself. I made plans to ask why I had not been chosen as a way of learning from the rejection. If I found myself doing a poor job while in the residency, I would ask for help and not see that as a sign of weakness, and I would tap into my network of faculty, friends, and colleagues for assistance.

The third step: Write down options of what to do if my fears came true. I reminded myself that chances of being selected were not on my side. I also knew that since I had completed a PGY1 residency in California, I had a high likelihood of finding a job if getting the PGY2 residency did not work out. I also listed my professional accomplishments to date and saw that I had achieved some success. Finally, I listed options for a change in professional focus, such as working for a pharmaceutical company, a professional organization, or community pharmacy.

The fourth step: Write down the positive consequences of success for both the short-term and long-term. If I did well in the administrative residency, I would move into management where I could grow and become a director of pharmacy, implementing new and innovative ideas for the practice of pharmacy.

The fifth step: Write down what would happen if I did not pursue the PGY2 residency and left things the way they were. I would attempt to find a job as a clinical pharmacist, which I knew I would enjoy. If I later wanted to pursue a management career, I would work in a setting that would allow me to progress up the career ladder through experience and further education.

This five-step process demonstrated that I had options not only in what my next job would be but how I chose to manage the options emotionally. I have used the same basic technique of processing fears and doubts throughout my life in personal as well as professional decisions. Although I have found the process helpful, it does not mean I don't lose sleep or worry. It does mean that I don't dwell on issues after I have written the answers to all the steps. I have learned to trust my decisions, take risks, and allow myself to fail. I believe "fear-processing" has positively affected my successes, outlook on life, and level of happiness.

Another opportunity for growth and learning that led me to face fears was taking my first management job right out of my PGY2 residency. I became an Assistant Director of Pharmacy at a 650-bed hospital in the Chicago area. I felt overwhelmed with the job and had concerns about not having enough time, skills, and knowledge to get all the work done. The long hours caused stress at home. I was constantly asking myself if I was I making the right operational and personnel decisions. The fear-processing technique led me to understand the importance of delegating, taking time for myself to recharge (I took up swimming), and networking at the state and local health-system pharmacy association level. It seemed as though I could not possibly find time for association activities, but I found positive consequences by learning from others and widening my network.

I was still improving my fear-processing technique when I gave birth to my son. I took on parenting as I did any project at work. Research what you don't know. It felt as though I had every book on child rearing on my nightstand. I thought I could follow in others' footsteps as I prepared and planned out how my son's childhood would progress. What I did not account for was that this little person had ideas of his own which did not fit into my plans. Becoming a parent has been one of the greatest joys of my life, but it taught me that life cannot be fully planned. I learned to be more pliable and take life's challenges as they come. The sense of responsibility and lack of time that came with parenting made use of the fear-processing technique more difficult but still worth the effort. The emotional investment that comes with parenting often exacerbated the perceptions that if a fear materialized, the results would be disastrous. I soon realized things were not as bad as they seemed, and disaster was not around every corner. I learned that when in a particularly high-stakes situation, your perceptions can be exaggerated. Over time, writing helped me minimize, if not eliminate, many of my parenting fears and doubts.

After many years in hospital pharmacy management, I was given the opportunity to change focus when a pharmacy colleague asked me to help him build a pharmacy consulting business. There were no references, and no continuing education courses to teach me how to do this. I had built my own consulting business when my son was young, so I knew how to set up and run a small business; work with marketing personnel; work from a home office; and work with clients, other consultants, and a board of directors. So, when I was asked to help grow the pharmacy consulting business in 2007 for a friend, I felt I could apply the same principles as before. Once I embarked on this venture, some fears and doubts unexpectedly bubbled up. I had concerns about working with a colleague and how we would get along. I wondered if my prior consulting work would bring the skills I now needed. These concerns were not as profound as they had been when I was younger. I used fear-reprocessing as I realized the same concerns do return. All went well as the consulting business grew.

No matter how big the challenge, by working through fears and doubts that potentially keep me stuck, I *can* find a way forward. We all have had opportunities for growth and learning in our lives. I hope you can be aware of opportunities that come your way by paying attention and being open to new experiences. I recommend that you take the time to go back and define what opportunities presented themselves and examine how you embraced them. Identify any fears and doubts and how they affected the outcomes from the opportunity. Go through this fear-processing technique and see what you discover. Have the expectation that the same or related anxieties will arise but know you will get better at recognizing them and working through them. I think it is helpful to visit your fear-processing writings from time to time. What applies in one situation may apply to others in your life.

I wish you all the best in your future and in your professional and personal journeys and hope you find the fear-processing technique helpful.

Kathy

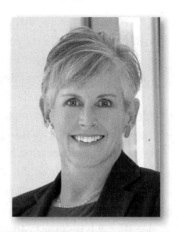

Leigh Briscoe-Dwyer
PharmD, BCPS, FASHP

The Value of Planning and a Personal Mission Statement

Leigh outlines her approach to being successful in both her career and life, indicating that success is something YOU define because you are in charge of your destiny. She also shares her unique #MeToo experience and what she has learned about working effectively with men.

Leigh is currently Vice President of Network Pharmacy, Northeast Provider Solutions, which is a member of Westchester Medical Center Health Network, Valhalla, New York. Previously she was Vice President, Clinical Affairs, PharMEDium Services, LLC, Lake Forest, Illinois. Leigh received her BS in Pharmacy (1987) from Albany College of Pharmacy, Albany, New York, and her PharmD (1994) from St. John's University, Jamaica, New York.

Leigh's advice is: Make a plan. Write it down. Consult your plan at least once a year so you are where you need to be to meet your goals. Reprioritize when needed, and don't feel bad about it.

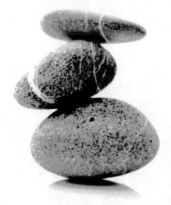

Dear Colleague,

It is said that "If you don't know where you're going then any road will take you there." This sage advice has helped me throughout my career. Make a plan. Write it down. Consult your plan at least once a year so you are where you need to be to meet your goals. Reprioritize when needed, and don't feel bad about it—your goals at 30 may, and probably should, be significantly different than when you were 20.

When I graduated from pharmacy school in 1987, the Doctor of Pharmacy degree was not yet entry level. I wasn't ready to go directly into a program, but I felt it needed to be part of my future plan. I also knew that once I entered the workforce and started earning money—*real* money—it would be hard to go back to being a full-time student. The goal I wrote down was to have my PharmD before I turned 30. Having that written down and being able to look at it every year was important because planning for something so significant takes time. I spent four years preparing for that goal—taking Master's courses I could roll over into the PharmD program, working a second and then a third part-time job to have money set aside for the two years I would not be working, finally applying, and then getting accepted into a program. I finished my PharmD program in May 1994, a few days before my 30th birthday.

Planning for a lifelong career may seem daunting—and to some it may seem presumptive—but it's really about perspective. You give time and attention to planning your wedding, deciding whether or not to have children, and buying a home, so why wouldn't you give the same priority to planning a career that you will spend at least one third of your life doing? If I had not developed a career plan, I would in all likelihood still be at the community hospital where I started my career 30 years ago. I was good at my job, I liked my team of co-workers, and there was enough variation in my job functions to keep me from being bored. However, after a while I did not feel challenged. I was getting too comfortable and was growing complacent about my work. To continue challenging myself, I needed to move to another job. To make the right career move, I felt I needed an advanced degree, and I was glad I already had my plan in place to make that happen. The same holds true of many important career or professional goals. We all want to practice at the top of our profession. For some, that means going back to school, passing a board certification exam, being promoted to a director of pharmacy, or being named a fellow of ASHP. All of these are achievable goals but ones that require planning, sacrifice, and time.

I developed a personal mission statement that I use as my compass when considering big life or career changes:

- I will be known as a devoted wife, passionate pharmacist leader, and loving and loyal friend.

- I will deliver on my commitments.

- I will continually improve myself by being a lifelong learner, staying true to my Catholic faith, and living a healthy lifestyle.

If the change in question will help me to fulfill that mission statement, then it deserves consideration. If it doesn't, then I may say "not now" and defer the change to another time.

The integration of work and life also requires planning and preparation. My husband retired several years ago while I continue to work, which makes for some unique challenges. I once read an article on the topic of working outside the home while your spouse/partner does not. The article advised giving the spouse an equivalent title in the family as you have at work and to treat him as such while you are at work. I took this advice to heart. Because I am the Director of the Pharmacy Department, then he is the Director of the Family. This indicates that he is as important to me as the rest of my colleagues. If he calls while I am at work, I will answer if it is not impossible—even if only to say when I will call him back. I print a copy of my weekly schedule for him so he has an idea of what my days are like. One of the downsides of this activity is that it becomes very clear when I have overcommitted myself and have left no time for our family. I find it helpful to block out evenings for "no appointments" well in advance so I don't find myself in that situation. Making your spouse or partner feel included in your work makes them more invested in your career, and I believe this increases your likelihood of success.

Remember that success is something that YOU define. You certainly need mentors and advisors, but you cannot judge your success by someone else's. By planning your own path and holding yourself accountable, you will realize that you are in charge of your destiny. Every successful person has had feelings of inadequacy because we are all aware many people are smarter or better or more qualified than we are. Use those feelings as a catalyst much in the same way you use the adrenalin that runs through your system right before a big meeting or lecture. Let those feelings sharpen your resolve and bring clarity to your role so you work with more efficiency and purpose. Remind yourself that health-care today is different and more dynamic than ever before, and old rules do not apply anymore. If you are uncomfortable as a leader then *you are doing your job.* Success, when it does come, will be that much more satisfying.

In the early years of my career, the majority of pharmacists were men. It is not surprising that my first leaders and mentors were men, and that I developed a management style similar to those who taught me. Now that women make up more than half of the new graduates entering the pharmacy workforce, I expect management styles will change to reflect the different ways women and men perform as managers. However, one of the biggest differences I have noticed as a manager is the style in which men and women deal with disagreements at work.

I have seen men argue—sometimes vehemently—at work. Voices will be raised, fingers will be pointed, and tempers may flare. I will see the same two men go to lunch together the next day as if nothing had happened. If two women had the same argument, they would often not speak to one another for weeks! I admit to often seeing this characteristic in my own interactions, primarily because I took things too personally.

Men seem to be better able to compartmentalize things at work and better at differentiating the "work" person and the issues at hand from the "whole" person. I once asked a male co-worker about his relationship with another male he had to let go due to performance issues. He replied that they still met occasionally for lunch, because he still liked him as a person. This ability to "fight like a guy" is a specific trait I learned from my male mentors, and it has been a great help to me.

The #MeToo movement has spurred much needed conversations around how women should be treated in the workplace. Interestingly, much of the back-stabbing and career sabotage I have experienced in my career has not come from men, but from other women. My decision not to have children was a conscious choice that I am perfectly content with. That does not mean I want to work every major holiday because I have no children at home. If I plan to come in an hour later than usual because I am training for a marathon and need to get my miles in, it should be treated with the same respect as if I had to attend a morning program for my child at school. If I earned a promotion, it is because I planned for it, worked hard for it, and aced the interview, not because the hiring director is a man who thought I was pretty.

As women, we need to do some reflection here and make sure we are not part of the problem. We must support one another in our career and family choices and rejoice in the success of our fellow women. The glass ceiling exists, so it is very likely that when a woman has a huge success or a great achievement she probably had to work harder and longer to get there. Celebrate her success and hope that someday soon that ceiling will become a lens through which the achievements of *all* people are seen in their truest and most equal light.

Leigh

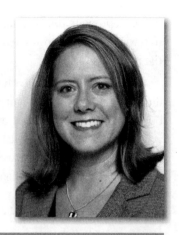

Angela T. Cassano
PharmD, BCPS, FASHP

Polish Your Perspectives to Clarify the Focal Points in Life

Early in her career, Angela formed her own consulting company, which has since thrived. A wife, mother, entrepreneur, and breast cancer survivor, Angela has been able to convert life's ambiguities and challenges into successes through her strong mindset and determination. Angela reflects on the curves and sharp turns in her life that required sharpening her focus on priorities, assuming risks, and maintaining a healthy perspective on the many roles she balances.

Angela is President and Founder of Pharmfusion Consulting, LLC. Throughout her career she has held positions as a hospital Clinical Pharmacist, a Clinical Assistant Director, and an Assistant Health-System Director of Quality Assurance and Drug Safety. She received her PharmD (1999) from Campbell University and completed postgraduate year 1 and 2 (PGY1-PGY2) residencies at Virginia Commonwealth University.

Angela's advice is: **We worry about many things that steal our time, passions, and energy. They shift our focus away from the gifts we have been given and wear us down. Refocus. Make the most of each situation. Learn from every opportunity.**

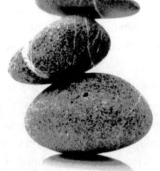

Dear Colleague,

When I initially submitted my letter I didn't write about my cancer journey, about my "something," largely because I have talked about it a lot over the years. For once I was asked to focus on Angela, the entrepreneur, not Angela, the cancer survivor. But a mentor encouraged me to rewrite my letter to share my story from the standpoint of providing hope for the next generation.

While my journey involves cancer, yours may involve a different type of life-changing scenario—divorce, death of a loved one, or a lay off. I talk openly, but there is always a part of me that is uncomfortable sharing my story. I never want anyone to assume that I think my road was harder than anyone else's. My situation was no better or worse, but perhaps I can make a difference in your journey by sharing how the lens in which I viewed my story shaped far more than my health outcome.

Before January 15, 2007, I was a wife, daughter, sister, and mother to a busy two-year-old daughter. I was someone of strong faith, and a fairly new business owner. My primary objective as a business owner was likely different from some people's—to be a mom first. I had supported my husband through his residency and fellowship, and I was ready to work part-time for a few years. My secondary objectives were to continue making a difference and staying relevant within the field of pharmacy so when I was ready to work full-time again I could make a smooth transition. I felt then and now that I was given a gift of education and training, and I was determined to continue using it to help others while first and foremost being a mom. To me it is the best of both worlds!

I started Pharmfusion Consulting in August 2005 with hopes of focusing on smart infusion pump implementation and optimization, along with sterile compounding training and auditing for USP Chapter <797> compliance. I had worked on the forefront of both areas and was excited to help others succeed. I was confident about my abilities and was sure that whatever I needed to learn about running a business I would figure out with help from mentors.

What I hadn't anticipated was that the demand in the marketplace called for most of the smart infusion pump and sterile compounding support to be done on-site. I went from being very confident to very confused about what I had to offer as a consultant. I had to adapt quickly and decide how to change my business model, and I had to be comfortable making a difference from behind the scenes and from afar. I began to evaluate my skills and was honest with myself about them.

I realized there were a lot of tasks I enjoyed that were likely not favorites of others, and I could do many of them from a distance. It was humbling to see that what I valued at this point in my career was very different from the aspirations I had as a new graduate. Then I had dreamed of one day having my name on the spine of a textbook. But I chose to step back from being a "rock star" clinician and accept that I'd be solidly alright crunching numbers in a basement office instead of being by a patient's bedside. It wasn't sexy, but it required me to see my world through the lens of what mattered most not just to me, but to my family. For me, it was finding the balance to help others and finding professional fulfillment while working from home on my own terms.

Fast forward to January 2007. Although I was making the most of the opportunities that came my way as a consultant, realistically, very little of what I had envisioned actually materialized; if it did, it required significant travel and time away from home—and both were counter to my primary goal. As one of my projects, I became the coordinator for a pharmacology and therapeutics course at a Master of Physician's Assistant program.

I was keeping long hours developing the course that started the first week of January. I will forever believe that was the stressor that brought my cancer to the surface. I was having numbness in my right arm and thought it was carpel tunnel syndrome. But a self-examination revealed a tiny lump in my right breast. Doctors' visits eventually confirmed an additional lump in my axilla, which was pressing on a nerve and causing the numbness. I was 31 years old and was diagnosed with stage IIB breast cancer. Overnight I embarked on a chemotherapy and bilateral mastectomy journey. Very quickly my world came into sharp focus, and only what was truly important remained. I was scared but had plenty of hope and a strong desire to not only come out the other side intact, but to make sure my business came out intact too. I refused to go through this trial and let it take away my goals!

It is safe to say many pharmacists are "type A"—we like detail, we like order, we expect perfection for our patient's sake if nothing else, and we have been trained to do it ourselves. Life-changing events throw all of that into chaos, and how well you manage the fact that you are no longer in charge has a significant impact on your journey. Certain things fall off the to-do list. For once in my life I was finally comfortable saying no to requests of my time. My body was broken. I was bloated and puffy due to the steroids. I was bald. I had scars all the way across my chest and will never appear normal in that regard again. But my spirit was not broken, largely due to my faith, but in no small part due to the network of colleagues, friends, and family who carried me along the way. My mother moved out to Ohio to help keep things as normal as possible for my daughter. They developed a special bond that remains to this day—just one example of a blessing from harder times.

Eleven years after my diagnosis, I celebrate each year not only as a survivor, but as a business owner too. This letter made me reflect on what has allowed me to achieve my professional goals. My projects for Pharmfusion are still largely done from afar, but now they are more closely aligned with my original professional goals of working on sterile compounding and technology. Many of my projects are for national pharmacist or pharmacy technician organizations, and each project expands my horizons and my ability to make a difference. I had originally planned to work two to three years as a consultant until my daughter went to kindergarten. She started high school this year, and I don't foresee working anywhere other than where I am right now. When I think about what made this dream possible, two words come to mind—networking and determination.

The first concept, **networking**, is something we are taught early in life. It is as simple as making friends—particularly the ones who will answer your calls. Yes, texting and emails may have taken over, but be sure to cultivate your relationships. Your professional network should be less about where people work or what they do in their work, and more about the quality of the jobs they do and the genuine interest they have in you as a person. Often your network is a grassroots effort that starts from natural places. It starts with classmates, professors, preceptors, alumni, co-workers, etc. Your network should continue to grow throughout your career as your interests change. The longer I work as a consultant, the more my network and track record have replaced my book knowledge and expertise as my most important business assets.

The second concept, **determination**, is simple in theory. You put your head down, don't take no for an answer, and brush yourself off when you fall. These clichés have been hammered out in stories that went before mine—but my journey has been no different. Perhaps the most important thing that cancer taught me about determination was that there are a lot of worries in life stealing our time, passions, energy, and focus. They shift our sights away from the gifts we have been given and wear us down as we run the rat race of our jobs and lives. Life-changing events demand a level of dedication and energy, which require us to let go of the trivial and reach out for help. They require us to reprioritize what is absolutely sacred and what can fall away. The challenge is to remember this once life hopefully goes back to "normal."

I wish I could say I am confident enough to not care what others think or worry about telling people no or not now, but I'm human. For me, survivor's guilt is a real thing and my world goes back to center every time another friend or family member loses their battle with cancer. In that respect I regularly ask *"Why me? Why am I here and they are not?"* I don't know the answer to those questions, but I do believe I have a responsibility to take each moment and be the best wife, mom, family member, pharmacist, business owner, and friend for the time I have. I am thankful for my network, both personal and professional, that saw me through dark times and got me to this place. And I am thankful I never let go of the goal to be a mom first!

Sincerely,

Angela

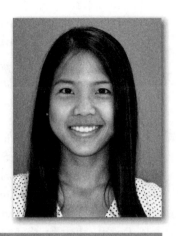

Sophia R. Chhay
PharmD

Life, Liberty, and the Pursuit of Leadership

As a first-generation female pharmacist, Sophia shares her personal story of how she broke through cultural barriers and family expectations to follow her own leadership pathway. Academic performance versus following one's own interests is an unspoken tension with many first-generation families. Asserting personal independence while also respecting parental desires and social norms requires a delicate balance but is necessary to grow into your own person.

Sophia is currently the ASHP Strategic and Innovative Initiatives Associate. She also serves as the Program Coordinator for the ASHP Executive Fellowship in Association Leadership and Management. Previously, Sophia was the ASHP Executive Fellow from 2017–2018 and a postgraduate year 1 (PGY1) pharmacy resident at the Erie Veterans Affairs Medical Center. She completed her PharmD (2016) at the University of Findlay College of Pharmacy.

Sophia's advice is: It is a beautiful and liberating aspect of life to be imperfect. Allow yourself to accept the gift of imperfection, and give yourself the freedom to take risks.

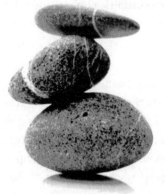

Dear Colleague,

I am writing this letter today on a very special occasion. It is Mother's Day. I cannot thank my mom enough for all she has endured and done for me and my siblings. I love her, respect her, and cherish her, but I did not always agree with her growing up. Being a first-generation Asian American comes with a set of challenges, particularly when you are a female. Please know that the story I am about to share is not about remorse, anger, or ill-will but, really, unconditional love, bravery, and resilience.

"Life, Liberty, and the Pursuit of Happiness" is the well-known phrase from the United States Declaration of Independence and exemplifies the unalienable rights of the American people. It is also the reason many immigrants, including my parents, sought refuge in this country. When Vietnam invaded Cambodia in the late 1970s, my grandparents arranged an escape from the war for each of their children. Both of my parents eventually made it to the states. My dad was the first one of his siblings; my mom was the last of hers. At best, I can imagine what this experience was like for them as I listen to the stories that are seldom told. Despite their firsthand accounts, I will never be able to truly understand the struggles they went through.

I realized later in life that this important history is part of the reason I was raised the way I was. As a child, I was told to do well in school so I could get a job that paid well. Good grades were valued highly and extracurricular activities were seen as unnecessary distractors. I should forget about having a social life because I was a girl, and girls should not be socializing or interacting with the opposite sex. In Cambodian, there is a term for girls like this—*srey swa*. My mom used to always tell me not to be a *srey swa* because it is the lowest way for a girl to be seen. I was obedient in virtually every aspect of my Cambodian culture except this one. I simply did not see extracurricular activities and socializing as a bad thing. I saw it as an opportunity, a learning and growing experience, a door to something greater.

Breaking cultural norms is no small task. Living in a household where respecting your elders is a hard and fast rule made it that much more difficult to be defiant. But I respectfully fought back. And in many cases, as you sometimes should in life, I compromised. Instead of going out for multiple sports, I went out for one. I was determined to give everything I had to the opportunities I was afforded. I became captain of my high school soccer team. In college, I was elected president of the women's club soccer team. In a way, I wanted to prove to myself that this was a worthy endeavor despite my mother's disapproval.

I made sure to maintain my high academic performance to appease her. However, as I sought additional extracurricular experiences, I had to compromise again. This time, it was with myself. If I wanted to continue participating in student government, my pharmacy fraternity, and professional pharmacy organizations, I was going to have to put in even more hours to keep my grades up— more hours than I had to spare. The question I found myself asking was, *"What was I willing to give up?"* I replayed this question over and over, hoping that the answer would pop into my head. Instead, the answer appeared in my heart. I didn't actually have to give up anything. I loved being engaged in my professional organizations, and I could tell I was becoming a better student, leader, and person for it. Thus, I allowed myself to accept the gift of imperfection.

Having high expectations for yourself is a good thing, but if they are unrealistic, that can be harmful. If we were always perfect, we would not be human. I wish I had realized this sooner because it is a beautiful and liberating aspect of life to be imperfect. As long as my GPA was above a 3.0, I decided that it was good enough. I allowed myself to pursue additional leadership positions and, as a result, I grew in ways both professionally and personally. Becoming a graduate assistant for continuing education for the college of pharmacy taught me how to embrace and foster lifelong learning even before I became a pharmacist. I served on the executive board of my Student Societies of Health-System Pharmacy (SSHP) and became the student liaison for the Council for Ohio Health Care Advocacy, which broadened my understanding of healthcare legislation and the impact of grassroots efforts. Through my leadership within Kappa Epsilon, I learned about recruitment, networking, and communications. Meanwhile, I was developing many soft skills—how to delegate, motivate, inspire, and brand myself. I also learned how to resolve conflicts and how to approach difficult situations.

In my third year of pharmacy school, I decided to apply for the ASHP elective Advanced Pharmacy Practice Experience (APPE) rotation and got to experience the inner workings of a national pharmacy organization. It's safe to say that I drank the association Kool-Aid. Indeed, I found my passion. I loved everything about my experience at ASHP. It was the perfect blend of the organization's mission, vision, and incredible staff that had me hooked. I thought to myself, I would love to work here someday!

During my PGY1 pharmacy residency, I served on the ASHP Council on Education and Workforce Development as the new practitioner member. Here was yet another volunteer experience that would require additional hours, but to me it felt less like work and more like another exceptional opportunity. I got to work and connect with many great leaders in pharmacy. Moreover, I got to be a part of something that was bigger than me. A majority of ASHP's professional policies are born in the councils. This was a rare and enriching experience for me as a young professional, and I was honored to be a part of it all.

My engagement with ASHP seemed to follow a trajectory as I was selected for the 2017–2018 ASHP Executive Fellowship in Association Leadership and

Management. I can still remember getting the call from Kasey Thompson, ASHP Chief Operating Officer and my program director. I could barely contain my excitement as I verbally accepted the offer. Throughout my fellowship, I worked closely with the ASHP senior leadership team on various projects and ASHP initiatives as well as received their mentorship in all facets of not-for-profit association leadership and management. As my predecessors would echo, this fellowship is a life-changing experience. It has stretched me in ways beyond what I thought was ever possible. I am thankful every day for the opportunity to have an impact on the profession of pharmacy, our members, and the patients we serve. There is no better feeling than loving what you do and making a difference. To me, that is true success.

As I wonder how to close this letter, I reflect back to how I opened it—with my mom. Today, she has told me countless times how proud she is of me and everything I have accomplished. I have shared with her how grateful I am for all that she has done for me and my siblings. I realize she sacrificed many things in her life so that we would not have to sacrifice anything in ours. I am living my American dream because of her.

My biggest hope is that you, too, have great, strong women in your life to look up to, lean on, and learn from. Further, I hope that we can join these women in empowering others and leading positive change.

Sincerely yours,

Sophia

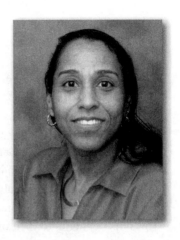

Marie A. Chisholm-Burns
PharmD, MPH, MBA, FCCP, FASHP, FAST

Why Pursue Leadership?

Marie is an excellent example of the value of education and the circumstances of your birth not defining who you become. Despite growing up in a town where the high school graduation rate was less than 30%, her parents—who had not attended college—were relentless in their dream for their only daughter to graduate not just from high school but also college. While growing up, they often reminded her of the adage, "*It's not how you start that's important, but how you finish!*" She credits a solid foundation of hard work, honesty, integrity, and giving back for her success.

Marie is currently Dean and Professor of the University of Tennessee Health Science Center College of Pharmacy and Professor of Surgery in the College of Medicine. She previously served as Professor and Head of the Department of Pharmacy Practice and Science at the University of Arizona College of Pharmacy, with joint appointments as Professor in the Department of Surgery and the Division of Health Promotion Sciences. Chisholm-Burns received her BS in Psychology and General

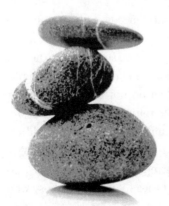

Studies (emphasis in Biology) from Georgia College, BS in Pharmacy and PharmD (1993) degrees from the University of Georgia, MPH from Emory University, and MBA from the University of Memphis. She completed her residency at Mercer University Southern School of Pharmacy and at Piedmont Hospital in Atlanta, Georgia.

Marie's advice is: **We need your influence and your leadership as well as your ability to inspire and influence others to help them achieve their goals, serve as a role model and mentor, and hold open those doors for others that I had to break down with a sledgehammer.**

Dear Colleague,

Although many of us may be able to cite the names of a few prominent women able to break the proverbial glass ceiling in pharmacy leadership, the overall percentage of women occupying key leadership positions, unfortunately, remains dismal. Regardless of sector, from academia to community pharmacy, not only is the number gloomy, but women in these positions are more often isolated and faced with challenges unaccustomed to their male counterparts. These experiences (some subtle, some blatant, all disempowering) often lead to women doubting their abilities and value, and even inhibiting them from pursuing leadership positions outright or from excelling to their full potential. This limits benefits to their organizations and the people they serve.

I personally understand how the lack of a critical mass of role models who resemble oneself, coupled with disparate treatment in the work environment, can discourage a hard-working and productive individual. However, I also understand how critical it is that we do not allow these deterrents, many of which are barely recognized or even acknowledged, to paralyze or defeat our ambitions to obtain the leadership positions that we so richly deserve and that our organizations need.

You may ask: Given the aforementioned frustrations, why pursue leadership? What makes this worth it?

My answer: "The ability to influence."

Specifically for me, it is the ability to inspire and influence others to help them achieve their goals, serve as a role model and mentor, and hold open those doors for others that I had to break down with a sledgehammer. Moreover, I believe that the improvements we need in education and healthcare can only be achieved through the inclusion and valuation of diverse perspectives, experiences, opinions, and aspirations.

There is no doubt that my background has influenced—and continues to influence—my actions and results. It is a fierce motivator that urged me to change my past circumstances and still urges me today. You see, I have witnessed society's scales of justice in newspapers; on television; in board rooms, committees, and various other settings. These scales often do not tip or balance for people who are different from those in power. Therefore, my relentless desire to work hard, uphold ethics, speak out against injustices, and make a difference were destined to be in my character as part of my environment and DNA makeup. I write this letter to the talented, underrepresented individuals who stand on the outside waiting for doors of opportunities to open—for those who want to make a difference and provide benefit not only to themselves, but to the organizations and professions they serve. I write this letter to these individuals who are considering the difficult but highly rewarding path of leadership.

As I reflect on my experiences in pursuing leadership positions, there are 10 key strategies that I have found particularly useful throughout my career.

I share this "prescription" to excel:

1. **Build a network of trusted mentors, sponsors, and cheerleaders.** Seek out this support and then pay it forward by being a trusted mentor, sponsor, and cheerleader for someone else.

2. **Develop a career plan.** Recognize and pursue the education, training, experiences, and skills needed to be successful in the desired position. Commit to it and put it in writing.

3. **Consider saying "yes" to challenging and visible assignments.** Identify and acknowledge that you possess the skills necessary to accomplish these assignments, and completing them will enable you to grow personally and professionally.

4. **Promote/market yourself.** Do not assume your good works will get duly recognized. Although you may leave it to others to discuss or even brag about your good works and talents, do not be afraid to appropriately mention your successes.

5. **Dwell in the possibilities.** Look for opportunities and important gaps to fill. For example, if there is some core service or innovation missing from the market and/or your organization, and if you have the knowledge or skillset to address this gap, consider pursuing that possibility. Fill gaps that will bring high benefits and rewards.

6. **Network.** Meet with others and engage in the field.

7. **Believe in yourself and stand up for what you believe in (including yourself).** Do not wait to be anointed. Actively pursue the success you desire. Also speak out against injustices of preset biases in position searches and sexual harassment.

8. **Do not be paralyzed and overwhelmed with guilt.** You may feel a little guilty about not being able to do everything, but recognize this is a natural feeling. We all know that we want to be there for every event, whether big or small. However, the simple fact is that you cannot attend everything. No one can do that, and we should try to shed those unrealistic measures and

expectations of ourselves, especially the guilt from this unviable expectancy. Remember: Prioritize! Put those big things on the calendar first and give them priority.

9. *Learn from adversity.* There will be difficult times, but use your stumbling blocks as stepping stones. Try not to stay down for long and always keep moving.

10. *Be courageous—being a leader takes courage.* You may not be 100% confident in every situation. Accept that: To grow you must step out of your comfort zone from time to time. Consider these times as growth opportunities.

In addition to the "prescription" above, I want to make a special mention of work–life balance. This is one of the most significant areas I've had to tackle as a woman in leadership, and I know it often poses a critical challenge for women interested in leadership roles. It took me greater than two decades of experience to understand that instead of focusing on work–life balance, we should strive for life–work integration. My integration process is ongoing, but I have learned some good practices that may be useful to others. For example, at the beginning of my son's school year, I reserve time on my calendar (schedule it in and make it priority) for special school events and days away from the office for mommy and son time. After known family obligations are scheduled, then I integrate work commitments.

To make this integration successful, you may at times need to get others involved. My family and I often have meal deliveries and occasionally use landscapers and cleaning services. Do not feel guilty about utilizing these services. Use them as often as you see fit. For example, I am just waiting for the right moment to spring on my husband that I would love to have a car service for long driving trips. Speaking of my husband, I do have great spousal support (which occasionally involves driving me to work-related events), and he is also a major source of inspiration. Because we both work full time, we share in household and parental responsibilities. For big time commitments, we plan months in advance, especially given my high travel activity. My husband is fully aware of my travel schedule and always gets a copy of my travel itinerary. We call and text each other often, when I am in town and out, and we are committed to being very accessible to each other and our son. As with our jobs, we keep promises to each other as a family unit. In my position as dean as well as my roles as wife and mother, I try not to overcommit (some days are easier than others), while always trying to over-deliver.

As technology advances, I find myself utilizing more tools to keep in touch. There really *is* an app for everything! Just ask my son, as I know his assignment grades before he does (his claim anyway) because of a wonderful app. My point is, please remember to invest time in achieving life–work integration; and be willing and flexible enough to continuously work with your family and friends to find helpful strategies and tools and make adjustments addressing your life demands, including your social and family life.

Earlier I addressed the question, "What makes this worth it?" I think the natural follow up is, "Is it worth it?"

Let me state unequivocally: "yes, absolutely!" Nothing I have done, aside from my family, has been so impactful and meaningful in my life as being a leader in academic pharmacy. Beyond the ability to influence, leadership roles have afforded me opportunities to interact and learn from patients, students, and colleagues across the country (and globally). I have developed lifelong relationships and gained so much.

Pharmacy and U.S. healthcare in general are ever-evolving. To keep pace with changes, overcome challenges, and provide excellent care to our patients—as well as optimal education and training to future pharmacists—the pharmacy profession needs energetic, innovative, intelligent leaders. We need your diversity, inclusivity, knowledge, creativity, talents, representation, and skills. We need your influence and your leadership. *We need you! It's your time, it's our time!*

Best wishes,

Marie

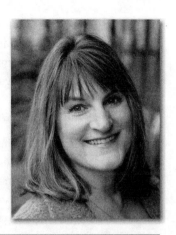

Cyndy A. Clegg
BS Pharm, MHA, FASHP

You Are Enough

Cyndy is a successful clinician and pharmacy administrator. She lives with integrity and a strong sense of professional commitment. Cyndy uses her sense of right to lead her through change and challenges. She shares her journey of finding self-confidence which includes getting rid of excuses, overcoming imposter syndrome, and stepping out with wisdom, experience, and having something of value to share.

Cyndy is currently the Director of Pharmacy at Swedish Edmonds Medical Center. Previously she was Assistant Director of Ambulatory Pharmacy Services at Harborview Medical Center. She received her BS in Pharmacy (1984) and MHA from the University of Washington.

Cyndy's advice is: **You cannot possibly know everything you need to know today. You must learn it through others—especially those who have been blessed with both successes and failures in life. Listen intently to their wise advice and learn from them, and don't doubt yourself! You are not a fraud or an imposter. You are enough. Winnie the Pooh said it best, "You are braver than you believe, stronger than you seem, and smarter than you think."**

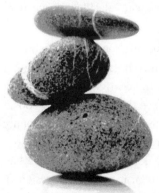

Dear Colleague,

The honor of being asked to write this letter gave me time to reflect on the negative perspective I once had of my abilities compared to how others saw me. How I wish I had felt that I was actually competent and successful! I struggled with writing this letter because, once again, I thought perhaps someone had made a mistake in choosing me to participate. I even missed the first deadline blaming it on writer's block. This opportunity has been a gift as I had to face my self-limiting beliefs and recognize I *am* worthy of my successes and achievement!

Let's Play Dodge Ball!

I was the awkward, frail, skinny kid in elementary school—the left-over student whenever captains chose teams in physical education (PE) class. I will never forget how the embarrassment and humiliation of walking slowly to the side stuck with me. It became a ritual over the years. They didn't even call my name; after the same girl was always picked right before me, I just walked to the other team. I wasn't chosen because I was a little weird and just wasn't good at sports, especially anything that required endurance. It wasn't until my twenties that the reason became apparent—I was finally diagnosed with a congenital heart defect so severe that I was living with a PO2 of 60. No wonder I couldn't run. Looking back, I think those weekly reminders of my skill deficits (some of which were health related) contributed to how I viewed myself and my capabilities in all facets of life.

Mom Always Knows Best

I grew up in a home with two working parents who didn't attend college. They made it crystal clear when I was very young that I needed to be well equipped for whatever life had in store for me. My mom told me countless times that I must have a career and be able to support myself. Although she and my dad were happily married, she was beginning to see the increasing divorce rate and women in the workplace struggling to support a family on one paycheck. She is 92 today, and we both still marvel at how these words of wisdom made such a difference in my life. With sagacious foresight from my mom and an introduction to health-care and pharmacy from my uncle, an anesthesiologist, I decided at age 11 to pursue pharmacy as my chosen career.

During my first 10 years of practice, I held three different jobs as an ambulatory pharmacist—I worked at a health maintenance organization, a hospital outpatient pharmacy, and a small community pharmacy. I changed jobs for a variety of reasons but looking back at my career, I see that in those early jobs, I was demonstrating the little *l* of leadership. It came pretty naturally to me; my very first pharmacy manager tried to get me interested in leadership in a more formal way, but I brushed it off thinking he was making a mistake. After I had been at one job for a couple of years, our outpatient pharmacy manager resigned.

I didn't apply or even consider applying for the job because I didn't think I had the skills and certainly didn't have the confidence, even though I functioned as the interim manager for nearly six months while we searched for a permanent manager. Lack of confidence? *Flashback: Elementary School PE.* Why would anyone want to choose ME to lead their team when those kids didn't even want me on their team?

I considered being a staff pharmacist as my only career goal. A leadership position never crossed my mind. If you had told me during my first year of practice that one day I would be a Director of Pharmacy, I would have laughed. In fact, if you would have told me as recently as five years ago that I would be the Director of Pharmacy for an acute care hospital, I would have told you that you were crazy!

Stop Making Excuses!

My next job was at a large academic medical center, and almost instantly I knew I had found my pharmacy home. I thrived in this environment, and I blossomed working for a nationally respected ambulatory pharmacy leader. But when a supervisory position opened up, I ducked. My lack of confidence and worry about measuring up found me making a lot of excuses about why I didn't apply; they included my family is my top priority, I'm pregnant, my life is complicated at the moment, I haven't got time, it's not exactly the job I want, I just had open heart surgery last year and I want to focus on my health, etc. All of these were actual reasons that I gave over the years!

Listen to Your Peers …They See You As You Really Are

When I finally applied for a formal leadership role, I was in crisis mode due to a crumbling marriage and desperately needed to make a change to survive. I had two boys: an 18-month-old and an 11-year-old and I realized to be successful at home as a single mom, I needed a different kind of certainty in my schedule. Working as a clinic-based pharmacist, I couldn't just get up and walk away from a patient appointment with daycare closure time looming. The trade-off was in deciding which I could best perform: a clinical role where I knew I needed additional study and the ability to stay late based on individual patient needs OR caring deeply for my team's performance and dedicating myself to their success in caring for patients. I was lost. But thanks to a colleague who encouraged me that I would be a great fit for the vacant leadership position, I marched into my manager's office immediately and said "now is the time." She welcomed me to leadership with open arms and incredible support. Although it was difficult to step away from direct patient care, I began to see myself using my innate little *l* strengths in a big *L* way to better serve the department and our patients.

Imposter Syndrome and Me

But oh, the doubt! When the inevitable challenges of being a new manager surfaced, I sensed the return of the shame. *Flashback: Elementary School PE.* The feelings of being a fraud and imposter crept in. Who am *I* to be leading this group of successful pharmacists and technicians?

It has been reassuring to read about "imposter syndrome" in the literature. I have always felt like someone was going to eventually find out that I was a fraud. It is estimated that 70% of us discount evidence of our abilities and feel like we aren't as good as others. In reality, our feelings of inadequacy feed our work ethic. We often set very high standards for ourselves and work very hard to achieve our goals.

Experiencing Mentor Magic

Although I can't blame it all on my elementary school PE experience, I see how those early years contributed to self-doubt and made me feel inadequate. Fortunately, there have been several mentors along my journey telling me a different story about my future than the one I was imagining. I vividly remember having dinner at the ASHP Midyear Clinical Meeting in New Orleans with my mentor, a respected leader and Whitney recipient. We were discussing my career, and he challenged me with, "What's next for you?" At the time I was a pharmacy supervisor working for an amazing leader—that perfect mentor/coach/role model for whom I had tremendous respect. I was lucky to be blessed with working for her (she would say WITH her) for 16 years. I thought her skills, knowledge, and abilities were so far superior to mine that I told him I could never step into her shoes. My mentor enthusiastically responded, "Of course you can!" Continuing our conversation, we explored why I felt that way, which eventually led to uncovering my overall lack of confidence and faith in my own abilities. His wise advice over bananas Foster led me to apply to graduate school. Returning to school for my Master's in Health Administration (MHA) paved the way for so many opportunities I never imagined for myself. This was a pivotal moment for me. *Listen intently when a demonstrated leader takes an interest in your career path. They have the wisdom, experience, and the long view. Heed the good advice!*

Back to School and the Best Boss Ever

The first day of my MHA program involved some serious team building on a ropes course. We spent the majority of the day in increasingly difficult exercises with our new classmates. The last challenge of the day found me in a five-point harness on belay, climbing 30 feet into a tree and jumping off a small platform. Standing up there, we were asked to state our intentions for graduate school. "Confidence" was the first thing that came to my mind. "I want to be more confident." My heart was racing, and I was anything but confident as I took the leap off that little piece of wood. During the two years of my MHA coursework, my manager served as ASHP President. She had the faith that I could represent our department when she was away for Board meetings and other ASHP responsibilities. While this was challenging at times, she trusted me to care for our staff and patients just as she would. Because I didn't do a residency after graduation from pharmacy school, I have jokingly referred to her presidential term as my health-system pharmacy administration residency. She encouraged me to become actively involved with ASHP. Wisely, I took that advice too. Because of her, I met her wonderful friends and colleagues who ultimately helped me to become actively involved in section advisory groups, Policy Week, and other ASHP committees. Those three years of her presidency, with her strong support and encouragement, as well as my studies were a huge turning point in the self-limiting view I had perfected. There was evidence of achievement and worth, and I finally started to believe it. Never mind that I was almost 25 years into my career at this point! A few months after completing my degree, she was promoted and I was promoted into her previous job—the one a mere four years earlier I told my mentor I could never do. When she retired, I was on my own. And all of a sudden, the phone started ringing and colleagues across the country would call and ask my advice. I remember hanging up the phone one day and wondering: *When did I become THAT person ... the one with wisdom, experience, and something of value to share?*

Stepping Out with Confidence

After 20 years of service, I left the academic medical center for a director position in ambulatory care at a local hospital system. There was a lot of work ahead of me to advance the retail pharmacy and homecare practice at my new job. I finally believed in my abilities as a pharmacy leader and my ability to positively impact the care of patients within this new organization. My entire career had been in the ambulatory world, and I was confident I would be successful in this next challenge. Then, eight months into my new job, the Chief Pharmacy Officer appeared in my office and asked me to consider adding the 200-bed inpatient pharmacy services to my span of control. ACUTE CARE? The last time I worked in an acute care setting had been at this same hospital 33 years earlier as a pharmacy intern! But guess what? That doubt? It lasted all of five minutes. I took a deep breath and remembered my colleagues, my mentor, and that best boss ever. I reminded myself that I am a work in progress. That accomplishing anything—including great things—takes a lifetime of experience and learning, even for the most confident people. I could "own" my success this time and spend my energy making a difference for patients and my staff instead of second-guessing my abilities.

The important lessons aren't in books or in the classroom. They come from others who share their wisdom, advice, and guidance that will light your path. Listen intently to what they have to say. I wish for you self-confidence, accompanied by hard work and a healthy dose of humility. Listen to your heart. And when you find your rhythm, enjoy marching to the beat. And whenever you get the chance, pay it forward.

All the best,

Cyndy

Lourdes M. Cuéllar
BS Pharm, MS, FTSHP, FASHP

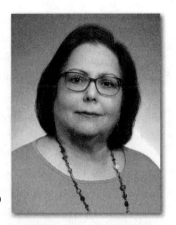

Breaking the Glass Ceiling through Passion, Perseverance, and Resilience

Lourdes, or "Lou," has been a long-standing leader at the state and national level. She has observed and initiated much change in the profession. As a Hispanic woman leader, Lourdes is passionate about supporting other minority women to assume leadership roles in practice and in professional associations. She encourages readers not to be defined by gender or ethnicity and to take risks that may be uncomfortable, such as speaking up, having those difficult conversations, or making a tough decision. The courage to do so may be leveraged by finding your own inspiration for change.

Lourdes is Administrative Director of Pharmacy and was previously Director of Pharmacy, Outpatient Medical Clinics and Clinical Support Services at TIRR Memorial Hermann in the Texas Medical Center. She is also an Adjunct Clinical Professor of Pharmacy Practice at the University of Houston and the University of the Incarnate Word. She received her BS in Pharmacy (1973) and MPA (1979) from University of Houston.

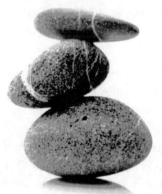

Lourdes' advice is: "Never let success go to your head and never let failure go to your heart."
– Zaid K. Abdelnour

Dear Colleague,

As I navigate the winter of my career, I have spent time reflecting on areas that gave me the most joy in pharmacy leadership. A topic that quickly comes to mind is continuously working toward improving the presence and recognition of minority pharmacy leaders, especially women leaders—an area that continues to be a critical weakness in our esteemed profession.

Developing talented minority women for leadership positions is no longer an aspiration but a fundamental necessity for our profession. *Why is this issue important? Where are these essential leaders?* Minority women who ponder questions such as why, when, or what if—along with visionary transformation goals for our profession—should make the commitment to take a step, even a small step forward in the direction of their passion and leadership goals. The importance of increasing the number of minority women leaders in pharmacy is far more important outside of political correctness.

I want to share a snapshot of my story. As you read this letter, I hope it will move you to embrace my message and continue the quest to change the face of pharmacy leadership.

I am a middle child, which brings its own recognized characteristics. I was very independent, quite curious, and mischievous, and made friends with everyone I encountered. I was always optimistic and ready for any and all adventures. My college experience was shaped by the events of the 1970s and by living at a time when there were quotas for minorities in many of the institutions of higher learning. This was also the beginning of the post-Civil Rights movement that inspired a desire by both Hispanic and African American students to bring the essence of their culture—for better understanding—to their college campuses. Many of us (minorities) carry hidden scars that framed our passions, perseverance, and resilience in life, family, educational, religious, social, and work encounters.

One of my first experiences as a female in pharmacy was working as a pharmacy intern in the VA hospital in Houston. My friend and I were the first two women ever to work in the department (except for the secretary). It was both amusing and enlightening to see the behavioral changes that occurred as we integrated into this very large male-dominated department. By the time we left after graduation, one of our female classmates would become their first female pharmacy resident.

Culture plays an important role in setting priorities for many women, and this includes my own Hispanic culture. Some ethnic cultures emphasize family over individual success. Males are encouraged to become successful and go into respected professions; the same conversations may not occur with the female children. The woman's priorities of raising and caring for family are stressed. I was very fortunate that my parents firmly impressed on all three siblings that we would go to college; we would succeed no matter what career we chose. In their eyes, it was a way out of poverty; an acquisition of knowledge could not be taken away from us.

Many strong minority women who have leadership aspirations make choices toward family responsibilities early in their career. Often when they are ready to join or rejoin the workforce, they will encounter other barriers. Many women overcome these barriers by keeping strong networking connections and continuing their self-development while making family a priority.

One of the core principles I learned early was developing a sense of purpose that was aligned with my personal and professional values. Characteristics that I have always admired in leaders are passion, integrity, humility, leading by example, active listening, and finding one's "voice." Many strong leaders that I work with every day do not have a formal title, yet they are remarkable trans-formational leaders. They display resilience, and despite success demonstrate a humble character. They are innovators, engage others in their vision, and recognize and give credit where it is due.

When I graduated from pharmacy school, my goal was to attain a residency and pursue a path toward pharmacy leadership and management. I was limited geographically where I could apply due to financial reasons, and I did not attain a residency position. After some reflection, I made the decision to continue on with graduate school and meet the practice qualifications through my position and through partnership training at neighboring institutions. After six years as a pediatric practitioner and an MS in Pharmacy Administration under my belt, I was given the opportunity to interview for a position as Director of Pharmacy. Thirty eight years ago, I was the lone female pharmacy director in the Texas Medical Center (TMC) in Houston. There have been other strong female leaders in the TMC who have served and moved on, but leadership positions to this day still seem to be held by men.

One of the obstacles I had to overcome was breaking into the "men's circle" during quarterly TMC pharmacy leadership meetings. Having a sense of purpose, addressing common concerns, possessing confidence in my leadership potential, and being committed to the leadership group helped me crack the glass ceiling. The men's circle became my colleagues and mentors, and our interactions were as peers. We all served as resources and helped to support one another.

A totally unexpected barrier encountered early in my leadership career came from other women. After several years as Pharmacy Director, I assumed responsibility for several other clinical departments within our hospital. Following my promotion, two female department directors asked to meet with me. The message both delivered was that they should have been promoted because they were older and had seniority from the standpoint of service to the hospital. My initial response was surprise, but I said that I understood their concern. I was honored to have been offered the promotion, and any discussion about their abilities and desires for promotion should be directed to the hospital administration. Both later apologized, recognizing they were directing their annoyance at the wrong person. *Would this question have been asked if it had been a man who was promoted under similar circumstances?* I had a similar experience when an opportunity arose for a leadership position at our national organization. Some pushback suddenly emerged from another female leader. More frequently than expected, it seems that women are barriers to success for other women. It is important for strong, successful women to celebrate and motivate other successful women and not find ways to undermine them.

Friends and colleagues know the quote that has always given me purpose in life and in my profession is M. Gandhi's, *"Be the change that you wish to see in the world."* This desire inspires me to take risks that may be uncomfortable, such as speaking up, having those difficult conversations, or making a decision because it is the right thing to do. It helps me to not let failure go to my heart and allows me to learn from setbacks and move forward.

Although I have been honored and privileged to be recognized as a leader in my profession, it brings added responsibility in that I also represent minority women. In my case, it is Hispanics, which constitute the smallest number by measured ethnicity of practicing pharmacists in the United States. My purpose has never been to seek out organizational leadership roles. I have always been driven to serve my profession and community and advocate moving our profession toward the top of our license. Active participation in pharmacy associations at the local, state, and national levels, as well as governmental appointments has afforded me countless leadership opportunities for which I am very grateful.

One of the more important roles I can fulfill as a minority pharmacy leader is recognizing and nurturing the leadership skills of minority pharmacist and technician colleagues. A question I have always asked at the end of employee evaluations is, *"Is there anything I can do to help you meet your goals?"* Once, I was asked what made me happy as a pharmacy leader. I responded it was when I see a colleague or a former student or resident succeed.

As a female minority leader, visibility and education of our future practitioners is a high priority. I serve as an Adjunct Clinical Professor of Pharmacy Practice and teach P-1 students the core principles of health literacy and cultural competency. Upon invitation, I also facilitate a MS/administration residency seminar on leadership and serve as a panelist in their Capstone course. In addition, for many years I have been the practitioner advisor for the Mexican American Pharmacy Student Association. I invite minority pharmacists to speak and interact with students about their respective areas of practice whether in leadership or as clinicians. It is important that students interact with minority pharmacy role models and understand early in their didactic training the immense opportunities they can aspire to beyond the traditional pharmacist roles.

Through the Texas Society of Health-System Pharmacists (TSHP), I have partnered with other leaders in providing leadership development for our members, especially young practitioners. As minority women leaders, we can model change by being strong, effective mentors for pharmacy students and residents. Being an active preceptor and engaging the students in leadership development can be successfully integrated into any experiential rotation.

Lastly, my brother (a life-long community pharmacist) and I have established scholarships at our alma mater, the University of Houston, College of Pharmacy and through TSHP. These scholarships were created to provide qualified students of Hispanic heritage with an opportunity to complete a pharmacy education. The goal of these scholarships is to promote academic excellence and to provide an opportunity for a student with financial need to reach their fullest potential. If there are no eligible Hispanic students, the scholarship is open to students of other minority heritage. I can think of no better way to give back to the profession than to provide opportunities for the next generations.

Although gender differences may exist in leadership styles of men and women, I have not experienced any difference in leadership effectiveness. When women attain leadership positions, they are successful. However, organizational change and mentoring programs that mirror education and acceptance are needed as minority professional women encounter far more difficulties in attaining leadership roles. I hope to see future leadership researchers address identity information such as gender, race, and ethnicity to help advance minority women toward pharmacy leadership roles.

The good news is that women in general are achieving leadership positions despite the barriers. Regardless of your job function, be the best at it. Do not let gender or ethnicity define the story of your career; let your dreams and passions define your career. Find and network with men and women, especially minority leaders who inspire you. Develop relationships that allow you to grow and excel. In the April 2018 *O, The Oprah Magazine*, Oprah Winfrey asks the question: ***"What are you willing to stand up for?"*** She continues, "There are countless ways to get loud about the topics you care about, or to stretch yourself beyond your comfort zone to make your message heard." I found my voice; what about you?

Developing talented minority women leaders is no longer an aspiration but a *fundamental necessity* for our profession. Promoting and increasing the representation of minority women in pharmacy leadership is the right thing to do. Create your own path; find your voice; find strong mentors and network; and encourage one another. Be willing to speak up because your voice matters! Courage is not born in a moment or a day—it is a journey.

Pick up your hammer and break the glass ceiling,

Lourdes

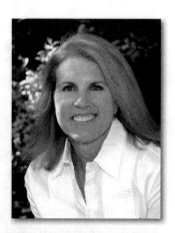

Debra Devereaux
BS Pharm, MBA

Be Flexible, Work Hard, and Be Nice

Deb is a pharmacist leader who prioritizes honesty and a direct approach to problem-solving. Deb is currently Senior Vice President, Pharmacy and Clinical Solutions, Gorman Health Group. In 2002, she served as ASHP President. Deb received her BS Pharmacy degree (1976) at the University of Colorado and her MBA (1986) at Regis University, Denver, Colorado.

Deb's advice is: Leaders can only be leaders if there are people following them. You can't be a leader if you never acknowledge that you made a mistake or if you can't change your mind.

Dear Colleague,

I remember my exact "aha" moment when I decided I wanted to become a phar-

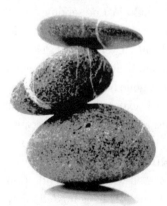

macist. I was a high school junior and had an after-school job wrapping Christmas presents at my Rexall Drugstore in Paonia, Colorado. The relief pharmacist was Theo Colburn who encouraged me to pursue pharmacy because of my love of science and helping people. She also provided a positive role model for combining work she loved and a family. I have had my fair share of these serendipitous, fortuitous, or happenstance occurrences in my life that allowed me to see a clear path which wasn't at first obvious.

As Dr. Seuss might have said, I have had an "Oh the Places You'll Go" pharmacy career while remaining in my beloved Colorado. I started in the pharmacy department at an academic medical center, moved to academia in a university school of pharmacy, and am now a consultant in managed care. In each of these organizations, I started off as a staff member and was promoted to a leadership role. I have found leadership to be 90% wonderful and 10% terrible. The 10% terrible is usually associated with crucial conversations with employees and/or colleagues that have negative outcomes. Most of these encounters are permanently etched in my memory—calling security to assist in removing an employee in the middle of a psychotic episode, confronting employees with substance abuse problems, and breaking up a fist-fight between two employees. The 90% is most often associated with a sense of accomplishment and the satisfaction of achieving goals.

I pride myself on being flexible. Each of my jobs positioned me to be successful in the next one. My successes gave me the confidence to assume more responsibility and to give myself credit. My Assistant Director position at the University of Colorado Medical Center and my work with the medical and nursing staff on the institutional review board (IRB), clinical pharmacy teams, and other hospital committees proved to be excellent training for my role in the school of pharmacy managing the drug utilization review (DUR) program. Understanding government regulations and being exposed to government programs positioned me for a consulting role at the beginning of the Medicare Part D program when no pharmacists had that skillset. I have a "Can I do this?" voice that I pay attention to, but my defense is usually to over-prepare so that even if I don't succeed at something it isn't because I didn't make the effort.

How did it all go? Sometimes the answer was not very well. Tragedy sometimes really is comedy plus time. I am not a big believer in work–life balance. **Balancing priorities** would better characterize my philosophy. My family, friends, and health are always in my top five list. It might just be sending a text or making a quick call to my kids, but maintaining connections to family and friends is crucial to socialization and good mental health. Exercise and sleep are fundamental to maintaining physical health and accomplishing all that is needed for your job and other responsibilities. My system has gone haywire many times. My children can relate times when I didn't meet their expectations. Mom-guilt is definitely a "thing." I could tell you lots of stories about getting sick because I ran myself completely off the rails trying to do too much. I recall one snowy February day when my pediatrician walked into the exam room and viewed my 4-year-old son, 1-year-old daughter, and myself—all with fevers and strep throat—and shaking his head said "You guys look terrible." I have missed many family events and disappointed friends because of misplaced priorities. I have to remind myself constantly to think before I say *yes* and commit myself to an obligation that will upend my priorities.

I have two children, and my pregnancies were awful—I had 9 months of morning sickness. My priority was trying to survive and maintain some semblance of competence at work. I had a couch moved into my office, and I worked laying on it sometimes. As soon as I got home, I went to bed and tried to eat and rest. I was also enrolled in an evening MBA program that had classes twice weekly. In retrospect, I don't know how I actually did it other than by basic determination. I graduated, and the kids were born—all in a 3-year period.

Another Assistant Director and I successfully convinced our Director to allow job sharing for a few years while both of us had very small children. This was before there were few job-sharing opportunities for managers. We committed to each working three 10-hour days weekly with one day where we overlapped. We communicated daily, covered each other for vacations, supported each other's decisions, and maintained this arrangement for about three years. I think the staff and our boss had some doubts, but because our management styles were similar, there was minimal disruption.

My husband's job necessitated a move to a smaller community in northern Colorado, and I applied for and was selected to be the Director of Pharmacy at a small behavioral health hospital that was to open the same month our house was finished. Then the hospital never opened, which obviously necessitated a change in plans. I worked part-time for several years at hospitals in Fort Collins and Denver until serendipity struck again. The Dean at the University of Wyoming School of Pharmacy called and asked me to interview for a new position as the DUR Coordinator for Wyoming Medicaid. I interviewed and was hired to manage the program, which was primarily virtual. I was usually in the office one day a week and managed the patient/provider database remotely, which turned out to be ideal with two busy school-age children.

Throughout my career, I have been involved with professional organizations in pharmacy. One of my first bosses introduced me to the local health-system organization as well as ASHP. I was elected to several state positions and volunteered for ASHP work groups and special interest groups, and was appointed to a council position and then elected to the ASHP Board of Directors. I had the ultimate honor to be elected President of ASHP and served 2002–2003. During Council week in 2001, the 9-11 terrorist attacks occurred. Steve Shaeffer was ASHP President, and I was President-Elect. It was a very difficult week with many council members stuck in Washington and unable to get home. The stories of planes, trains, and rental cars ferrying council members home across the United States are equal parts awe-inspiring and funny. I received so much more than I ever gave with my service to ASHP. The wonderful colleagues who I met, the leadership experiences and the knowledge gained, and the places I traveled to comprise one of the most amazing experiences of my life. Those colleagues are life-long friends who I continue to cherish.

I have not felt that being a woman caused me to be discriminated against in pharmacy—at least 99% of the time. In an interview for a Director of Pharmacy position, the physician interviewer asked me how I was going to handle my soon-to-be-born child and the job. I thought about telling him that it was an illegal question but decided to just reply that I wouldn't have a problem. We ended up moving 6 months after that, so probably not getting the job was for the best. I don't think many women my age have not been in some situations where there were improper remarks, insinuations, or generally boorish behavior. Depending on the situation and setting, I either ignored the person or confronted them. My first boss was fired for sexual harassment after complaints from two of his administrative assistants and an investigation. On occasion, I witnessed his behavior to others and told him it wasn't appropriate, but I wasn't personally targeted. I believe there are instances of harassment or discrimination where you must be fierce and refuse to tolerate behavior that is threatening to you. The current #MeToo movement is long overdue for many industries and professions in our society.

My credo would probably be **work hard and be nice.** I strive to demonstrate loyalty, integrity, and tenacity to get the job done. In management, you don't always "win" your positions. It's not that your positions are wrong, they just may not be timely, affordable, or congruent with the organization's priorities. Over my career I have learned the hard lesson that you can't control what other people do or think. You can only control *your* attitude and how *you* react when people or situations fail to meet your expectations. I recently was denied budgetary approval for several requests that I felt were very important for the success of my practice areas. Although I was disappointed and irritated, the entire organization's goals are the primary consideration and I had to accept the decision. Realistically, I know problems are not solved in the middle of the night; however, I still have some 2–4 a.m. sessions where I wrestle a two-ton problem that actually weighs two pounds.

Leaders can only be leaders if there are people following them. I have never been reluctant to jump in and get my hands dirty whether it was making an I.V., counseling patients, or working with challenging clients. I think teams have more respect for those who lead by example. You can't be a leader if you never acknowledge that you made a mistake or if you can't change your mind. As part of a recent performance evaluation process, I asked my managers what they needed from me that they weren't receiving. I value honest feedback, and I got it. One told me that I didn't provide enough positive affirmation for a job well done. He is right. I generally trust that when my staff is given assignments they will complete them, and the reports and deliverables will be high quality and meet client needs. I have taken the feedback to heart, and I am making an effort to ensure that when my staff performs well, I let them know.

Finally, I feel blessed to have had all the opportunities and experiences—good and bad—that made up my pharmacy career. I have few regrets and a store-house of wonderful friends and memories.

Warmest regards,

Deb

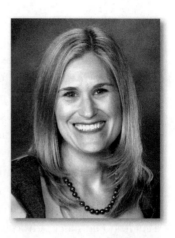

Lea S. Eiland
PharmD, BCPS, BCPPS, FASHP, FPPAG

Rejection, Failure, and Mistakes Occur at All Career Stages but Persevere

Lea projects an innate leadership presence, which spans from her student pharmacist years to her service on the ASHP Board of Directors. She is someone who epitomizes success. Yet, Lea opens up about her experiences with rejection, mistakes, and failures. Lea shares personal and practical advice on persevering through tough times and reflects on the people and experiences that continuously shape her determination.

Lea is a Clinical Professor and Associate Department Head of Pharmacy Practice at Auburn University, Harrison School of Pharmacy, and a Clinical Professor of Pediatrics with the University of Alabama at Birmingham School of Medicine, Huntsville Regional Medical Campus. She received her PharmD (2001) from The University of Texas at Austin and The University of Texas Health Science Center at San Antonio, and completed a pediatric specialty residency at Texas Tech University Health Sciences Center.

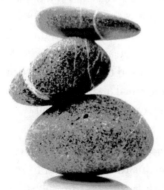

Lea's advice is: After a rejection or failure, it is OK to step away from the situation. Reflect, develop a new strategy, and then tackle it with determination. You may want to re-focus your efforts or ask a colleague to assist in order to reach your final goal.

Dear Colleague,

As you progress in your career, you may find yourself thinking that senior practitioners and leaders know the answers to all questions, can manage all projects, do not make mistakes, and are successful in every endeavor. However, that is not the case. At any stage in your career, you can and likely will experience rejection, failure, and mistakes. I have been a full-time faculty member for more than 15 years, and many people may describe my career as successful. I would agree that I have had successes, but I have also had challenges, failure, and rejections, and I am only mid-way through my career. *How recent you may ask?* Well today, I made a social media slipup, and last week I was notified not to submit a revision of a manuscript unless we (as authors) could satisfy every reviewer comment, which was not going to occur due to a philosophical difference. However, I also had one of the highlights of my career this week with the publication of the *ASHP-Pediatric Pharmacy Advocacy Group (PPAG) Guidelines for Providing Pediatric Pharmacy Services in Hospitals and Health Systems*, which I worked as part of team to develop for years. Despite the challenges, failures, and rejections, I keep going. *Why? Because you just do.* You learn from these situations, become more knowledgeable, stronger, wiser, and better as a pharmacist, teacher, mentor, and sponsor and usually the lesson trickles into your personal life as a wife/husband, daughter/son, granddaughter/grandson and, in general, as a person.

Determination and an optimistic attitude are key factors to accepting and moving on from these challenges, failures, and rejections. If you do not try, you will fail. *Now, how do I feel when these bad situations occur?* I feel like everyone else—mad, upset, embarrassed, frustrated, not valued, not talented enough, ____ (you fill in the blank), etc. *Do women react differently from men?* I think it is individualized. Sometimes you have to step away from the situation before you can analyze it and tackle it again. This break may be minutes, days, weeks, or even months. Once, I waited three months to work on a manuscript again after rejection. It took me that long to get to a positive place and start with a new mindset. I have found that if I tackle the situation immediately, I usually think of a better plan a day or two later. Emotions are not as strong, and I think more broadly about the situation. This is challenging though, as I usually want to solve the problem and move on to the next agenda item of my day. However, through experiences, I am reminded that a quick response is not always best. A male attendee at a conference stated that if he did not read—in the first sentence of an email—that his paper was accepted, he closed the email and would not open it again until Friday. He did not want it to affect his week of work. We all react differently and that is OK.

How do you move on and work through challenges, failures, and rejections? Everyone has their own method for working through situations. I tend to rely on ice cream and Thin Mint cookies! Then, I take time to reflect on the situation, including self-reflection, even after the situation is resolved. I may verify thoughts and gather feedback from colleagues. I determine what I can and cannot control in the situation. Sometimes I ask a colleague(s) to join in on the project. A multitude of ideas, perspectives, and hands can elevate a project as well as allow you to help others reach success. As you move along in your career, you will find that helping others succeed is just as or even more rewarding than your own success.

Speaking of success, you may ponder how those more seasoned professionals are successful. *What is their secret?* Did they have more than 24 hours in a day or not sleep at night? Surely, they did not have all the simple patients, easy projects, and friendly co-workers. *There is no secret.* Success is what you define it as and it may be personal, not professional goals. I have learned we all have the same hours in a day, similar challenges in the work environment, and personal activities that require our attention each day.

What characteristics contribute to success? There are so many but three key characteristics of successful people are ***prioritizing, planning,*** and ***perseverance.*** You have to ***prioritize*** your day to achieve the needed outcomes, plan for future outcomes, and keep focused on your goals. Every day, we all deal with the "fires" that arise during our normal responsibilities. Some days I accomplish a lot and mark off one key or many items on my to-do list. Other days, I have no idea what I completed but was busy all day. Really, watch how technology takes time away. Many leadership books recommend focusing on one task when arriving to work without checking email until a later time. Think about where you spend your time each day—you may think you know, but for one week write down your actions and then determine the priority of those activities, and see where you spend the most time. This may help you re-focus your time and be more successful with patient care responsibilities, project completion, meetings, etc. There are times when "no" is the best response. Also, remember you have and need personal time to do whatever it is you want, time that is not pharmacy-related. I make sure my Saturdays in the fall are planned around ESPN's GameDay. Growing up in Texas, I experienced first-hand Friday night lights and became an avid college football fan. I also enjoy reading and when I place reading as a priority, I achieve more balance in my day, especially when it is non-pharmacy/non-leadership reading!

Planning is also key. I am usually evaluating various outcomes that could occur with a project and activities or plans that need to be made in the future. A colleague tells me I am always thinking three to four steps ahead in the current plan. This allows me to strategize my time and efforts to assist our department and my personal objectives. It is critical to think of the implications of each decision that is made and how it affects the unit as a whole down to each involved individual, patient, or learner. Lastly, do not give up on your goals but be cognizant of when it is time to move on.

Persistence leads to success, sometimes in ways you did not expect. However, there are times when a goal may become unreachable. I have manuscripts that have never made it to publication. I tried many different ways to reach the goal before recognizing it was OK to stop and transition to another project. My time and efforts were best spent moving on.

Constant challenges we all experience are perceptions. Someone perceives he or she works hard, but others see a lack of work. Stereotypes of others are formed. Perceptions can influence our behaviors and feelings. After receiving an associate department head position, I was told by the department chair that some faculty members were concerned I would not be able to relate to them because I did not have children. Personally, I thought it was ironic since I am a pediatric pharmacist and at that time spent the majority of my day in the hospital with children. I understood they get sick, go on field trips, and require time of their parents or caregivers. I was once a child with a working single-mother. She was not able to come get me from school if needed, and we did not have family nearby to help. In this discussion with my department head, I told him that I felt I would be able to understand and empathize with situations related to children, even if I did not have one myself. *Would the same concern have been stated if I was not a woman without children?* My thought is *no*. At eight years in this role, this perception has never come up in discussions about my performance so I feel I demonstrated this was an inaccurate perception. Although it may be best, I find it extremely difficult to forget about others' perceptions of what you do or do not do. I believe it is important to recognize perceptions and think about how to change them if you do not feel they are accurate.

Our early developmental years shape our lives in many ways. My husband once told me that the apple fell off the tree and did not roll, when comparing me to my grandma and mom. When I think of my upbringing, I describe my grandma, mom, and me as three independent, single women. My mom is a retired teacher/principal who raised me. My grandma is 101 and was living independently until recently, as she now needs in-home assistance. She drove until a few months after age 100 and worked every Monday in the gift shop at the local, rural hospital until that time. She survived the early death of her husband, raised two children, and taught school. She was still a leader in her professional and social clubs in her 90s. I still recall when I realized in pharmacy school that she was born before penicillin. She was born at home and was the first of her siblings to go to college to earn a degree. Most of us will never see the amount of change she experienced in her lifetime—electricity, indoor plumbing, television, computers, and smart phones. I have always wondered how she does it. *How does she make it through failure, rejection, and challenges?* Determination, resilience, grit, fortitude, gratitude, an extremely positive attitude, acceptance of reality, and her faith. She is the one who taught me how to make it through life's difficulties. I can still recall when I called her in pharmacy school thinking the world was ending because I did not make a good grade in a course. She talked me through it, put it in perspective, and today she chuckles when reminding me of the call. The world did not end, and that grade did not affect my success in our profession. Several of my characteristics as a leader (as well as the importance of college football) come from my grandma and mom, my two women leader role models. *Who are your women leader role models?*

Our profession is not easy. Life is not easy, and it does not get easier as you age. We all experience failure, rejection, and challenges in our professional and personal lives at all ages. However, we can all make it through these situations and be successful. As my grandma reminds me, "This, too, shall pass."

Sincerely,

Lea

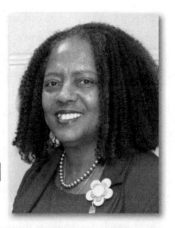

Vickie L. Ferdinand-Powell
PharmD, MS, FASHP

Each One Teach One

Vickie's lifelong love of learning and growing was stimulated by family members, educators, and friends who saw her leadership potential. Surrounding herself with good mentors, she moved rapidly into leadership positions while cultivating many enduring friendships with those who guided her and young people who were fortunate to receive her guidance. She encourages others to go beyond the path you envision for yourself and remember to invest in others who you see as a future leader.

Vickie is currently the Site Director of Operations at New York–Presbyterian Hospital. She received her BS in Pharmacy (1979) from Xavier University, her MPA (1993) from Long Island University, and her PharmD (2018) from Howard University.

Vickie's advice is: Adopt the motto "Each One Teach One." If each one of us could teach one other person, leadership will be sustained. Mentors must understand and appreciate their privileged position to support current and future leaders.

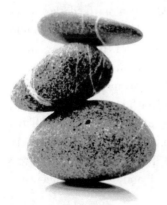

Dear Colleague,

The great scientist Albert Einstein revolutionized the way we view time, space, and gravity. He became a paragon of scientific achievement despite an impoverished background. To all great scientists who preceded him, Einstein expressed gratitude for the many contributions that enabled him to do so much in his chosen field. Like Einstein, I grew up in a poor family with meager resources and very little support. My father died when I was five years old, and my mother worked long hours as a domestic. After doing hard physical work each day, she had little time to spend enjoying life. My mother did not graduate from high school, and her family could not afford to send her to college. However, she always stressed her desire for me to get an education so that I would not have to work as hard (physically) as she did.

Her vision for me was to be the best at whatever I decided to do and to use my brain to make a positive impact in our community and the world. My mother also encouraged me to travel widely and seek experiences that were not available to her. She was my biggest cheerleader along with my grandmother who helped raise us and always encouraged me to be the best I could be. I am the first in my family to earn a college degree. My mother died one year after I graduated, so I was very lucky to have mentors who joined my extended family and inspired me to go further than I ever imagined.

I am truly a living testament to the power of mentoring. If it were not for my mentors' generosity of spirit, rigorous efforts, and the much-needed constructive critiques, I would not be where I am today. They provided leadership, education, counseling, friendship, and a professional roadmap for my success. They made learning fun, were always there to provide guidance, and after recognizing the tiniest spark in me, helped turn it into a flame. Sandra Day O'Connor, the retired Supreme Court Justice, once said, "We don't accomplish anything in this world alone, and whatever happens is the result of the whole tapestry of one's life and all the weavings of individual threads from one to another that create something." As leaders, we must be committed to mentoring and grooming others. The circle of life begins with learning, then continues with leading, teaching and finally, mentoring.

At an ASHP meeting, I had the honor of hearing a keynote lecture by Dr. Maya Angelou who shared the words of a 19th-century African American lyricist, Blind Andy Jenkins. "When it looked like the sun wouldn't shine anymore, God put a rainbow in the cloud." Dr. Angelou added, "Even on the darkest days, there was light." As I reflect on my growth in the field of pharmacy, I fondly remember my first mentor, Harvey Maldow. He was one of the rainbows in my cloud. Harvey and his wife, Renee, always provided caring advice and treated me like a daughter. He spent countless hours talking to me about the importance of making a contribution and getting involved in the New York State Council of Health-System Pharmacists (NYSCHP) and ASHP. As part of our benefits package, Harvey made sure funds were included for each pharmacist to join. During his presidency at the state level, he appointed me to committees with other seasoned pharmacy leaders in the Council and used his influence to advance me in the State Council.

Harvey also encouraged me to move into a management position and approved full funding for my Master's degree. He was my guide at ASHP and introduced me to influential leaders on a national level. His life lessons are ones I still use today. For example, Harvey taught me to remain flexible and open to the many changes one faces in life. He encouraged me to visit my staff regularly, hear their issues, and work collaboratively to solve problems before they escalated. His best advice was, "The problems will not come to your office. You must go out and hear them firsthand." He still checks up on me, and when he visits twice a year from Florida, we always get together

Two other rainbows in my cloud were Eric Hola and Michael Blumenfeld. Eric and Michael took me to high-level meetings at the hospital and made sure I met the most influential people in that community of professionals. These two colleagues set up opportunities for me to give presentations as the pharmacy leadership representative, which helped expand my knowledge and advance my career. We were like close siblings. I attended a Seder, Bar Mitzvahs, Bat Mitzvahs, and weddings for all of Michael's children. Each Easter for 25 years, I attended a Polish breakfast with Eric Hola's family and close friends. I especially remember how he made everyone feel as if they were the most important people in his life. We often talked at work, and I became a member of his extended family. Eric and I continued to speak by phone and have dinner updates until his death in 2015.

He introduced me to Lynnae Mahaney when I was appointed to a Council committee. She and I hit it off immediately and became close sisterly friends. I was honored when Lynnae came to New York to install me as President of the NYSCHP. I am sure my introduction to her resulted in an appointment to several other councils and committees on a national level. My husband and I became extended members of her family, and we had a special bond with her mother. Lynnae spent many hours sharing her professional knowledge with me and introduced me to many ASHP leaders. At national meetings, we always spent hours together sharing ideas.

Alan Cohen once said, "It takes a lot of courage to release the familiar and seemingly secure, to embrace the new. But there is no real security in what is no longer meaningful. There is more security in the adventurous and exciting, for in movement there is life, and in change there is power." His quote is reflective of my move from Supervisor at a small hospital to Director of Pharmacy at a large academic medical center. This change was a direct result of networking. It was never my intention to move into such a big role. My presidential induction speech at the New York City Society of Health-System Pharmacists installation was about the power of mentoring and how it helped me achieve things I never imagined. After that speech, the Apothecary-in-Chief, Karol Wollenburg, asked me to apply for an open director's position at her institution. I never dreamed that I would be picked as a Director of Pharmacy. Karol saw a spark and became the newest advisor in my rich treasure trove of mentors. She shared her vast knowledge with me, and I am now in my sixteenth year as Director of Pharmacy. I've loved every minute of it.

After serving as an administrator for many years, I felt a need to refresh my clinical skills. Two years ago, I decided to go back to pharmacy school to obtain my PharmD. My decision to go back was not because of a desire to move up in my career. I loved what I was doing, and I already had all the needed credentials. I went because the little voice that has driven me throughout my entire life spoke and said, "You can do it." And I listened. I am so thankful to the many people who helped me reach another milestone. I challenge you to adopt the motto, "Each One Teach One." If each one of us teaches one other person, the rainbows will be sustained forever, and we will have unlimited success. Mentors must understand and appreciate their privileged position as quiet, but engaged observers.

President Barack Obama once said, "The thing about hip-hop today is it's smart, it's insightful. The way they can communicate a complex message in a very short space is remarkable." When I was installed as President of the NYSCHP in 2009, my son wrote the following rap about mentoring, and I still treasure it today:

> Nobody does it alone
> Even a King is born a prince
> and has to learn how to handle
> the throne
> The way has to be shown by
> those who walked that road
> Somebody may have helped
> you to lighten your load
> Somebody must have done it
> for them
> So now that you're in position
> don't ever forget
> Each one teach one encourage
> their spark
> That's the best way to open a
> mind and open a heart

I'm so grateful to my son and daughter, David and Veronica, both of whom sacrificed the most during my career advancements. Throughout this long journey, I've been extremely fortunate to have my loving husband, David Powell, right by my side. He has supported me in countless ways. When I had doubts, Dave would say, "You can do it," and when I had success, he was the first one to say, "I'm so proud of you." Dave has been a rainbow in my cloud and my biggest cheerleader.

Vickie

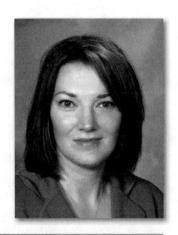

Erin R. Fox
PharmD, BCPS, FASHP

Say Yes to the Yes!

Drug shortages and skyrocketing drug prices have elevated Erin's authoritative voice into Congressional testimony, the *Wall Street Journal,* and *The New York Times.* Yet if you meet Erin, she is the last to seek a personal spotlight for any of her advocacy work. Erin has learned how to channel her knowledge into a powerful voice through her professional passions and from the support and encouragement of others. She has been able to achieve all of this by setting her mindset to "yes."

Erin is the Senior Director of Drug Information and Support Services and Program Director for the postgraduate year 2 (PGY2) drug information residency at University of Utah Health, as well as an Adjunct Associate Professor at the University of Utah College of Pharmacy. She received her PharmD (1999) from the University of Utah.

Erin's advice is: **Don't be afraid to say "yes" to opportunities that may be inconvenient.**

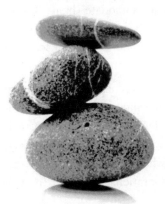

Dear Colleague,

How often have you received the advice to "learn how to say no"? Blogs, books, colleagues, and mentors advise prioritizing opportunities and thinking before you say yes. Magazines devote entire sections to "learning how to say no." I can't deny that's good advice, particularly when trying to balance children, marriage, and career. I can tell you that I've spent years always feeling guilty for saying "yes." I love my family, but I also love my job. I've missed soccer games, concerts, recitals, and even birthdays for different opportunities. I've spent a lot of time feeling terrible about myself not only for missing these events, but also being excited about the work I was doing that required missing those events. Recently, I decided that it's actually OK to feel this way. For me, I believe it's been a key to my personal success. It doesn't mean that I don't still feel guilty, but I've realized what a gift I have with my professional calling.

I have been blessed with extraordinary opportunities during my career. I had excellent training and mentors, the opportunity to work in a progressive organization, the room to grow into a leadership role, and the gift of working with the best colleagues bar none. Early in my career I volunteered to lead a new project to provide national drug shortage content. At the time, I was the newest staff member at our drug information service, yet I craved the opportunity to help fix what I thought was a frustrating situation for clinicians. I had no idea the project would mushroom into what it is today. At the same time, I was somewhat overwhelmed with the national audience for this work. The realization that my colleagues around the nation would be able to use information I provided to help patients at their organizations was really powerful. I knew I wanted to put my best efforts into this work every day.

As the drug shortage problem grew, opportunities to speak to the media came my way. My first reaction as an introvert was "absolutely not!" I hate being on television. I don't need to be in the news. I really don't want to worry about what my makeup and hair look like, or if my clothing will work on camera. I resisted being a part of the story, until the situation became so dire with the heparin shortage of 2008 that I decided the correct story was more important than my discomfort with media attention. I decided to say "yes" to reporters and make time for interviews. Over time, I gained the trust of many reporters, and they gained my trust by accurately reporting what I consider a public health crisis. Today I consider every request and try to accommodate them all—not because I want my name in *The New York Times*, but because I want the public to know that clinicians are forced to spend hundreds of hours each year sourcing basic products for our patients.

I won't lie to you and tell you that saying "yes" always ends up with everyone happy. Saying "yes" has meant hundreds of early morning and late night work sessions and plenty of tears and anger from my family (and myself). One particularly vivid memory was my first trip away from my oldest daughter. I had agreed to present at the ASHP Midyear Clinical Meeting while I was pregnant. I was so excited; it would be one of my first national presentations. I thought the trip would be fine since my daughter would be about 4 months old by the time I had to travel. I had absolutely no idea what I was agreeing to! I had no idea how traumatic it would be for me to leave my infant and travel across the country. My daughter was in absolutely no danger. My husband took great care of her and had the help of two sets of grandparents. Even though I knew she was safe and well cared for, I have almost no memory of that trip except crying while pumping and dumping every 6 hours. *Lesson learned.* When my second daughter was born, I had a volunteer opportunity that required attending a national meeting. Once again, I was so excited. I really thought the work of this group (ASHP Section of Clinical Specialists and Scientists) could make a difference for pharmacists and pharmacy practice. I thought about saying "no," but mainly thought of ways that I could say "yes." For this trip, I convinced my mother and my sister to take some vacation time and come with me. During the day they watched the baby, and we spent the evenings all together. We all had a wonderful time, and I count that trip as one of my fondest memories.

Saying "yes" can have some pretty strange side effects. In my case, I have learned that saying "yes" can result in almost paralyzing self-doubt. I took my first formal leadership role when my second daughter was just one year old. Rationally, I knew I could lead our drug information service. This was what I trained to do, and I had been an informal leader of our team for years. I also knew that I had an incredible support system with my husband and our parents. I also had the support of my team and key stakeholders. I had an ideal child care situation with a top program next door to my building. Still, I doubted myself constantly. *Did I truly deserve this position? Would I be able to be as successful as my mentor whose position I was taking? What would happen if I destroyed everything she, I, and the rest of our team had built?* To this day, I still doubt myself. Even though I have grown in our organization and have had the opportunity to take on more responsibilities, I always wonder if I truly deserve the position. After a recent promotion, I shared this doubt with a good friend who simply laughed at me and shook his head. He said he had never felt that he didn't deserve one of his promotions. *Lesson learned.* Even though I still have doubts, I try to embrace this philosophy that a promotion is almost certainly earned and well-deserved.

One of the most important lessons I've learned about saying "yes" is not to be afraid of inconvenient timing. Some of the very best experiences I have had are the result of saying "yes" despite knowing the timing was going to be difficult. When presented with the opportunity to testify for the Senate Aging Committee on drug prices, I had basically one afternoon to write my testimony. I had to say "yes" very quickly and completely redo my ASHP Midyear travel arrangements to skip much of the meeting and be in Washington, DC. Recently, I have been collaborating with a group of physicians from the DC area writing research papers about drug shortages. Over the past several years, we've published multiple reports, and I can tell you that in none of these cases did I have time to work on those papers. Each one resulted in hours spent during weekends and evenings crunching data and writing summaries. I would not trade those extra hours spent without sleep because I am so proud of this work that helps to raise awareness.

I mentioned I recently decided that saying "yes" was actually OK. This realization didn't come overnight, but instead slowly over the past several months. When a resident asked recently what one of my challenges was, I started to give my stock answer of "I have a hard time saying 'no' and end up overcommitted." However, as I gave that answer, I also mentioned that if I always said "no" if the timing was inconvenient, then I would have missed out on some amazing opportunities. I realized I wouldn't trade those opportunities for anything and that I truly can't imagine my life if I hadn't tried to always say "yes."

I hope my story will help you if you are feeling reluctant about a new opportunity because of timing, or have ever had doubts about taking on a new role. It's OK to say yes.

Remember, you deserve the opportunity or promotion!

Erin

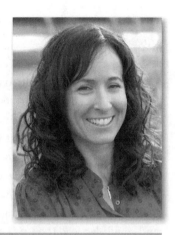

Dianna Gatto
PharmD, BCPS

Build Your Team, Build Your Career

Dianna finds energy and satisfaction from working with teams and describes how her leadership and success have been strengthened through team-building. Dianna is currently Clinical Pharmacy Manager and Pharmacy Residency Director at Multi-Care Good Samaritan Hospital in Puyallup, Washington.

Dianna graduated with a BS Pharmacy degree at Washington State University College of Pharmacy and received her PharmD (1998) from the University of Washington School of Pharmacy. Dianna completed an ASHP-accredited pharmacy residency at Good Samaritan Hospital, Puyallup, Washington.

Dianna's advice is: Find what gives you energy at work and what takes it away. Contribute no matter your role. Speak up. Your ideas and opinions matter. Find your teams, and if they don't exist, create them!

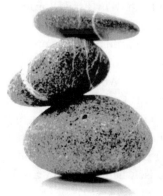

Dear Colleague,

What gives you energy at work? What takes it away? You should give these questions serious consideration. As I reflect on my career, what keeps me energized is *teamwork*. I have been fortunate to be a part of high-functioning teams throughout my career, from my pharmacy team to my home team. Surrounding yourself with people who give you energy leads to both personal and work satisfaction. *Learning how to identify and change what takes energy away gives you power.*

By knowing yourself and the answers to these questions, you control your life and career.

I started my pharmacy career by being the first resident at my institution. As an intern, I had learned to trust and rely on this pharmacy team. I had to trust that the program would meet the requirements for accreditation and obtain accreditation once I completed the year-long training. Likewise, the pharmacy team had to trust me—trust that I would be a model resident, an active participant on the team, and a good representative of their efforts. I had to engage preceptors, take and provide feedback, and follow through. This was challenging at times, as developing a new program requires lots of communication, engagement, and paperwork. During this process I learned that I worked well on a team and could also lead the team. I developed and used my motivational and communication skills to ensure preceptors had all rotation information completed and that we were "on the same page." Our teamwork led to the program's successful accreditation three months after I completed it.

Transitioning to my next role as a clinical pharmacist, I became a part of several teams—pharmacy, nurse, and provider. On each team, I learned the importance of developing and building trust. My high standards, strong work ethic, reliability, accountability, and contributions helped to build their trust. These teams trusted my knowledge and skills, and I trusted their abilities and feedback so that together we provided the best care for our patients. In each of my clinical areas, I forged strong relationships, which gave me energy and helped me be a better pharmacist and leader. In turn, the feedback I received was incorporated to develop myself.

As a clinical pharmacist, I never saw myself in a formal leadership role. I loved taking care of patients and working with acute care team members. After my residency, I had been asked to consider an administrative residency, but I hadn't considered it at that point in my career. I loved being a clinician and working directly with members of the healthcare team. *Why would I want to take on a leadership position?* A number of years after my residency, an opportunity arose to apply for a clinical management position and residency program director. Although the residency director position interested me, I didn't think about applying because management wasn't on my radar. When co-workers and supervisors encouraged me to apply, I was surprised, as I never saw myself in a leadership position. But, always being up for a challenge, I applied. I thought it would be a good experience, since it had been a while since I used my interview skills. I didn't have any expectations of obtaining the position because other candidates had more experience. Imagine my surprise when I learned I got the position!

Going from direct patient care to a clinical leadership and residency director challenged me. I hadn't developed clear plans or goals for myself or my team. My role on the pharmacy team changed overnight, and I had to reevaluate what this meant. I was no longer just a team member, but a leader and a coach. I focused on building trust and being transparent with my intent, especially as I was now the boss of former peers. I had a history of accountability with the team, but the rest was uncharted territory. If I said I was going to complete a task or project or follow up on a concern, I needed to follow through. This can be challenging in a management position due to numerous competing priorities. I felt compelled to do everything and felt guilty delegating to my team, because I knew they worked hard caring for patients. What I didn't realize at the time was that by taking everything on and owning it all, the team felt excluded. They wanted to contribute and to know their efforts were important and valued. Don't we all? Once I learned that, I had to take a step back because my intent certainly wasn't to exclude them. From that point forward, I changed my view of delegation and began including the team in decision-making.

At first, I found delegating difficult, even knowing how important it was for the team to contribute and for their contributions to be valued. It was hard because I didn't know how to delegate and wasn't always clear in my expectations. I didn't realize I had to consider an individual's strengths and weaknesses, which meant that sometimes projects were assigned to those who didn't have the right skill, interest, or ability. Not being clear with expectations meant the completed project often needed rework. The end results were numerous outstanding projects that required revisions and coaching, which I found slightly overwhelming. However, I learned from my errors and failures. I began setting clear expectations, assigning projects based on individual strengths, and pairing team members up for projects. The results are completed projects that meet my expectations, have team buy-in, and require few revisions.

Now, the team is my salvation. They are the reason I enjoy coming to work. *Did this happen overnight?* No, it didn't. It took a few years to build a strong team and to build my skills as a leader, and I'm not done yet! I built the team by capitalizing on our residency program and recruiting and hiring residents who were the right fit and had the same goals and vision as the team. In turn, these residents provided invaluable feedback to the continued development of our residency and preceptors. It was important to listen to and develop preceptors to promote our team, our residents, and each other. We hire pharmacists with a team focus and mentality. Learning from failures, listening to the team, being transparent, and being trustworthy enabled me to further develop my leadership skills.

My team gives me energy. Their focus in helping each other achieve excellence is inspiring. They not only let me know what obstacles they find, but they contribute ideas on how to solve problems. The team is aligned and focused on doing what is best for patients. In addition, they hold me accountable and provide open feedback. I find energy in supporting my team and removing barriers so they can provide optimal care to patients. Even though I don't see the immediate, direct effects of my work the way I did when I was a clinician, I am proud of the team, knowing the great work they do every day.

The most rewarding part of my job is building and maintaining teams, and the trust that allows this to happen. I want to be the best and want my teams to be the best. Working with teams is where I excel, and I have developed successful ones by following through and being accountable. To me, accountability means many things. It means owning my work, owning what I don't do, following through, owning my decisions, supporting them with logic, as well as setting and communicating goals and expectations while holding others accountable. It means listening to and incorporating feedback from the team, learning, adapting, trying new things, and admitting when I am wrong or make a mistake. I believe these characteristics have been instrumental to my success and have allowed me to create and be a part of highly functioning teams.

I share my expertise with residents and new pharmacy managers by providing lessons learned and advice so they are more likely to get it right the first time. It is essential to help them develop trust with their teams, learn what accountability looks like, and listen to the team, while keeping it all in perspective. The great part about mentoring is that I also benefit, not only learning from new leaders and residents, but by being reenergized through my teaching and coaching. These amazing new leaders support, encourage, and inspire me. They help me improve and grow.

My most vital team is my home team—my husband, two sons, parents, family, and friends. Together they support and rely on me. To give my best to my teams, I can't focus on only one, but must balance all. This can be challenging at times. *How do I give my best to everything?* Balancing work and life can be hard; with a strong work ethic, work can take priority, even when I don't intend it to. My family understands when work is a priority but also support personal time so I can de-stress. Find your outlets and know they may change over time. *How do I de-stress?* Exercise for me is key; currently that means running. I can leave work behind by focusing on my breathing and steps. My family also holds me accountable—when I need a break or am overwhelmed, they tell me. It's important to have people in my life who care and are invested in my well-being, who hold me accountable to taking care of myself.

When I think of where I have been and where I am going, I continually ask myself the following questions:

- What do I contribute to my teams?
- Who do I want to be?
- What attitude do I bring?
- What are my strengths?
- What are my areas for improvement?

Reflecting on these questions is important. Since teamwork is important to me, I want to contribute to all my teams. I do this by optimizing strengths and pairing myself with those with different strengths. Consider your strengths, what you contribute, and how you can improve. Teamwork makes me a better person and leader—no matter what my role. *What I have learned through this journey is that a team always makes better decisions than an individual, a team is more likely to get it right the first time, and a team makes challenging work fun.*

My advice to you is *find what gives you energy at work and what takes it away*. Contribute no matter what your role is. Speak up. Your ideas and opinions matter. Find your teams, and if they don't exist, create them! Everyone benefits from high-functioning teams; but most importantly, our patients benefit.

Good luck on your journey!

Dianna

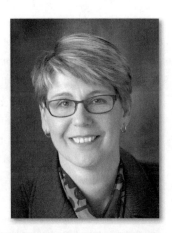

Christene Jolowsky
BS Pharm, MS

Sharing Our Common Focus as Women Pharmacists

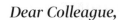

Chris is an active pharmacy leader at the state and national levels who shares her experience and wisdom; she is most proud of serving as the ASHP President in 2014. Chris is the Director of Pharmacy at Hennepin Health Care in Minneapolis.

Chris graduated with her BS Pharmacy (1981) and MS degrees from the University of Minnesota, and completed a two year ASHP-accredited residency at the University of Minnesota Hospitals and Clinic.

Chris's advice is: "If your actions create a legacy that inspires others to dream more, learn more, do more and become more, then, you are an excellent leader" — Dolly Parton.

Dear Colleague,

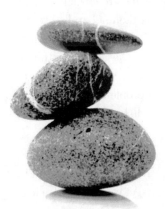

How are you doing? That is how I started my letters when I was young, when letters were written by hand. We have computers now, and part of the art of writing is gone as is the fun of receiving letters by mail. My next sentence was usually "I hope your family is doing well." I began my letters in that manner because it got me started. More importantly, it established that I cared about the receiver.

So, how are you doing? As a fellow woman pharmacist, I assume you have a myriad of details, large and small, running through your mind and probably a surplus of items on your plate. Sometimes this may energize you, other times it may overwhelm. So take some time to think about what is energizing and what is overwhelming, and I'll address this by giving you some advice.

My first piece of advice: Take it. Or leave it. Everyone has advice to offer. I found that advice often is a matter of timing and reflection. You can seek guidance to help clarify your options but, in the end, you need to make your own decisions and live with them.

Take pharmacy school, for example. I started out thinking I would be an actuary. My aunt and uncle convinced me to look into pharmacy. It was a good career for a woman, as it was possible to work part time and raise your children. So I considered pharmacy, but not to work part time. I liked chemistry and math. Although talking with a few of my classmates, I'm surprised I got in. This wasn't because of grades or references. One dean tried to persuade women applicants to consider home economics instead of pharmacy. If he had proposed that to me, I would have given a few choice words back, after getting over the shock. I found that pharmacy was a satisfying career for me, and it matched my skills and interest. There wasn't a single correct choice, but I made a good choice. Oh, and oddly, I have never worked part time.

I was active in PDX pharmacy fraternity during pharmacy school. That was interesting—the year I joined was the third year they allowed women. I ruled out joining Kappa Psi as women weren't full members, and the idea of being a "little sister" turned me off. Being a woman in the frat wasn't too bad, other than dealing with a few members who preferred to act like "frat-boys" rather than pharmacy students. It was tougher when I ran for vice-president and then president of the chapter. I became the first woman president of our chapter and the second in the nation for PDX. For most members, there were no issues with gender and my taking a leadership role. The frat-boys liked to challenge me. I'm not sure if it was because I was female or if it was just them. I handled some of the interactions fairly well—especially when being verbally challenged during meetings. I had plenty of opportunities to practice responses. I was confident in my role and responsibility and had other members on my side. I also practiced biting my tongue. **My advice:** If you can anticipate a problem, find people who will support you and ask them to be vocal. They can help buffer others who may get in the way, so you can do your job.

Like most students, I interned in pharmacy school. I worked at a hospital as a courier, technician, and then an intern. I often finished my assigned work first and then I helped others. At times it became a game to get work done efficiently, such as making sure that the credits were all put away and ensuring the area was cleaned up for the team on the next shift, which put them in a good mood. This was seen by others as my having a good work attitude, a willingness to go beyond my job, and working for the good of the team. *My advice:* Focus on both your assigned tasks and other tasks that need to be done as well. You're a smart person. Figure out where you can help.

Mentoring was not a common concept during my time in school or at least we didn't talk about finding mentors. I was fortunate to have a director who saw potential in me. He recommended I pursue a residency and Master's degree, which I did. I am grateful for his direction, a step which opened doors to the rest of my career and showed me a path to be a role model for others. My director is still a good friend and my biggest fan. I look forward to seeing him at our meetings, with a smile on his face and kind words. I thank him for the opportunities he showed me. *My advice:* Keep your fans close. They are the rays of sunshine on dreary days and help you stay energized about life. And just as your skills and talents are recognized, take time to recognize others.

Many of my girlfriends have stories about discrimination due to being a woman. I haven't experienced blatant discrimination, except once. Early in my career I interviewed with a company that contracted pharmacy management services. I was told the position was not good for a woman—too much travel and being away from home. I was stunned and didn't have a good response. Now, I would respond that I understand the job requirements and I am highly qualified for the position. Instead of this position, I accepted an assistant director position at a large hospital, had some incredible experiences for a first job out of school, met life-long pharmacy friends, and started on my way to organizational involvement. Oh, and that interviewer's concern about too much travel and being away from home too much? Maybe that was a premonition for what was in store for me as ASHP President. *My advice:* You will not get every position you apply for, and that is the way it is. Sometimes it turns out for the better.

My career has taken me to a wide range of settings, from very large hospitals to small systems, along with full-time and part-time consulting work, and academia. I made moves for various reasons, but never for the money. In one instance, I took a decrease in salary. Crazy? Not in the scheme of things. In my roles I've always had a good salary, and there is more to work than what you are paid. Pay also varies by location and position. I always felt that I was compensated commensurate to my position and responsibilities and in comparison to others in the organization. That's important. It is good to negotiate the best salary you can, but there may be limitations. If you are comfortable with the salary you accept, then go with it and remember that is your choice. You may find out information later that causes you to seek a higher salary, but, in general, be satisfied with your decision. Otherwise, it will be a thorn in your side. You may turn your focus on what others are making versus your responsibilities.

I have been overwhelmed with commitments. I often say "yes" without knowing the full impact of the request. Projects and positions often take more time than I thought they would, and a voice in my head then says "well, you thought wrong." A wise boss of mine said that the only way to get out of a hole was to stop digging. When I am overcommitted, I step back, focus on the work, lose some sleep, and move items off my plate to get out of the hole. Sadly for me, when I finish a few things, I realize I have time to do something else. *Lesson learned?* I don't say "no" well. I keep my commitments and have learned to accept requests in my areas of interest and expertise that keep me engaged.

Some things are present throughout your life and can't be moved off your plate. That includes your family. I have two wonderful, strong, confident daughters who are heading out in their own directions. As a mother, there were a lot of decisions that my husband and I made regarding raising a family. One was about day care. For our oldest, we connected with another couple and shared a nanny in our home. Raising our child and dealing with our own commutes and schedules was eased by our daughter staying in our home. For our second, we didn't find acceptable day care. After long discussions, we decided my husband would care for our daughter. He "stayed at home" for the next 14 years, and currently works part time. There were many adjustments, in terms of finances and household duties. In addition to being a caregiver, my husband picked up my part of the chores—so he did the yard work, cooking, and the laundry. He found he needed to be more organized during the day, and I found I needed to be accepting of what his day was like versus mine. We took about a year to settle with the changes. We found many "comforts" we could forego, which were replaced by a less hectic life. Having a full dinner on the table is not a luxury in our home—it is a nightly event. His biggest issue? Convincing others that this was a choice, and he was not just 'out of work!' *My advice:* You have a lot of decisions to make. Focus on what is important. In this case, it was our children. The choice was a good decision that allowed us time to focus on important parts of our lives and our family.

You will be told to find work–life balance. My work is more than my day-to-day job. I am a pharmacist, which I don't separate from my life. As I've grown in my career and in my commitment to professional organizations, the time demands have increased. Through the ups and downs in life, I've stayed involved in organizations, which gives me energy. I enjoy meeting up with my colleagues. I enjoy discussing challenges and projects and seeing others grow in our profession. My involvement has taken me from the local level to become President of ASHP, which I hold as one of my cherished accomplishments. *My advice:* Find your own balance. Life isn't equal.

We are all given 100%. No more, no less. This plays out in all areas such as athletic talents, intelligence, focus, attitude, behaviors, and interests. While my 100% is different than yours, we share the commonality of being women in the pharmacy workforce. As part of my 100%, I feel it is important to support and encourage other women. I have seen women promote themselves but not other women. As a grad student, I reached out to a prominent woman practitioner and author to discuss issues women face in pharmacy practice. Her response was "What? I don't have a problem." That was disheartening. Not that she didn't see a problem, but the response was belittling. I have also seen women who will come up with reasons why someone isn't deserving of recognition versus sharing their joy. I don't have much jealously in my 100% make-up. I will cheer on others and their accomplishments. I may reflect on what I could do to achieve the same recognition, but I am honestly happy for others. I have a history of being in leadership positions, and I feel it is important not only to be a role model to others, but to identify the talents in others and invite them to be involved and pursue new avenues. No matter how busy I am, no matter what else is going on, there is always time to recognize and acknowledge others. *My advice:* Celebrate accomplishments and don't let others steal your joy.

So my friend, I congratulate you on picking up this book and reading a letter or two or all of them. And when I ask "How are you?," I really would like to know.

Your fellow woman pharmacist,

Chris

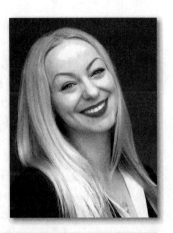

Sharon Karina
PharmD, BCMAS

Are You Ready for the Call?

Writing from a student perspective, Sharon provides insight into the stressors and competitive culture that student pharmacists face preceding and during pharmacy school. She reflects on the definitions of leadership and how difficult circumstances in life can force the development of leadership skills. It is increasingly important for student pharmacists to recognize and refine leadership skills so that they can be ready to assume their professional responsibilities upon graduation.

Sharon is currently Director of Educational Development at ProCE. She received her Associate of Science in Pre-Medical Studies from Triton College and her PharmD (2018) from Midwestern University, Chicago.

Sharon's advice is: All pharmacists are leaders, regardless of title or experience. Decisiveness, emotional intelligence, and vision are qualities many of us have that can be honed and developed to scale change.

Dear Colleague,

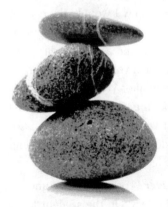

I still remember the moment when I first heard that I was a leader. Several weeks after a team-building exercise in my first semester of pharmacy school, I received an email from the faculty showing our secret rankings. I had been unanimously voted the leader of the group. *What does that even mean?* I filed it away, not knowing if it was an accomplishment or if I had been too eager to delegate and direct. The next three years of pharmacy school would lead to an awakening, reticence, and finally, avid acceptance of the word *leader* after looking outside and within.

Growing up in a single-income military household, I learned early in my life that happiness and success had to be fought for. Although we were blessed to always have a roof and electricity, I was helpless to solve our family's ongoing financial issues at my age. I sought refuge in school and was placed into gifted education. Unfortunately, circumstances outside of my control prevented me from graduating high school. I am a high-school dropout, and while I did receive a general equivalency diploma (GED), I was essentially treated as if I were a failure by others. I recognized that I had a choice to make about my life: either I could wallow in being a victim of circumstance, or I could objectively evaluate the situation and find another move to make. This was my first brush with decisiveness and a continuing influence as I managed life's challenges.

By all accounts, I should have never made it to college. Neither of my parents pursued higher education, and it was not financially feasible. It was difficult to not feel depressed, so I analyzed my family situation and looked at it from my parents' perspective. Perhaps it was a combination of lack of mentorship and finances that affected and influenced their story. I spent my early twenties working in customer service and longing for something more. During my marriage to my now ex-husband, I was able to self-fund my college education while he provided basic necessities. Decisiveness kept me going during the recession and led to my scholarships. My life has primed me with the ability to commit to decisions in times of crisis or uncertainty, and I have unknowingly developed a useful skill that, at the time, felt soul-crushingly unfair. As a woman, that decisiveness and drive can be misconstrued as the B-word. I heard that a former classmate, who I did not know, said my divorce was not a surprise because I was too career-driven.

Pharmacy school was not without its challenges. As my personal life was shaken to the core, I needed to start thinking about how I would take care of myself. It was then that I took advantage of my school's leadership development program. We were provided with an assigned mentor, and a mentor directory with contact information for all who were willing to be involved in the program. I reached out to all of them. What was your journey like? What are your challenges? **What advice do you have for someone like me?** Little did I know this would lead to an opportunity with Desi Kotis that was in part due to an Associate Dean's remark about me. And so began my deep dive into understanding what a leader was, and perhaps why others saw me as one.

What do you think of when you picture a leader? For me, it was someone with an earned title such as a director or vice president. On the student level, perhaps a student organization executive board position or a position in Rho Chi. Because I was not in a leadership position or had a title, I passively allowed others to speak on my behalf and kept filing the comments away. As I continued networking with others who had those titles, I began relating to the qualities that I defined for a leader: decisiveness, emotional intelligence, and a vision for the future—qualities I felt I had and could easily extrapolate from my own experiences throughout my life. Speaking with accomplished women at conferences reinforced my own experiences of the negative aspects of these qualities, as well.

Emotional intelligence was another aspect of leadership I deeply related to. Because I had actively decided to reason through some of my more unfair experiences, I relied on empathy to bridge the gap between differing opinions. I developed the ability to listen to other people and uncover their underlying concerns or problems. I began creating study guide content to help friends sift through important points in therapeutics and volunteering with a nonprofit organization, One Million Degrees, to give back to junior college students who also faced impossible financial difficulty pursuing higher education. I sat down with patients struggling to control their diabetes because of poverty and offered solutions within their reach to make lifestyle modifications. The downside of my empathy was the connection I built with some patients. I saw and experienced how unfair life can be in the faces of the dying and the mentally ill and the incredible barriers to care that lack of coverage or inflated costs create in our country. I hope to be a part of the discussion to change it.

I have a vision for a future that does not exist yet but could if we collaborate with the best minds to approach measured, evidence-driven goals. We are at a point where we can influence the direction of pharmacist leaders and create momentum to tackle some of our largest problems. I maintain that all pharmacists are leaders, regardless of earned titles or experience. Simon Sinek defined a leader very simply: *a leader is someone who has followers*. At the end of my academic journey, I realized I had my own followers who advocated for me behind the scenes, believed in my ideas, and gave me the opportunity to be heard. Leadership is not power or always earned by a title—it is a beautiful collaboration between many to achieve the impossible. Decisiveness, emotional intelligence, and vision are qualities that many of us have that can be honed and developed to scale change. I wish you all the best on your journey, from student to seasoned leader and everything in between.

Warm regards,

Sharon

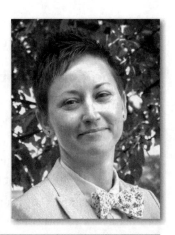

Lindsey R. Kelley
PharmD, MS

Vulnerability Is Courageous

If you have the pleasure of meeting Lindsey, you can sense her leadership presence through her confidence. The surprising key to Lindsey's confidence is actually through her vulnerability. Lindsey offers her advice to others about the importance of being authentic and open, and courageous in all that you do.

Lindsey is currently the Director of Ambulatory Pharmacy Services at Michigan Medicine, where she previously served as Assistant Director. She completed her BS in Chemistry (2001) at Northern Arizona University, her PharmD (2005) at University of Arizona, and her MS (2008) at University of Minnesota–Twin Cities.

Lindsey's advice is: Choose the hard thing. Be uncomfortable. Be vulnerable. Be courageous.

Dear Colleague,

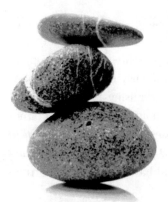

As I began to think about what advice I would impart to women pharmacists, I questioned whether I could identify anything worthwhile. I wondered aloud to my wife and colleagues: *Who am I to give advice? Do I have anything worth talking about?* And it was in asking those questions that an idea for this letter came to life.

Questioning ourselves is something we often do—we question our value, our ability to contribute, our worthiness. This has been a personal struggle for me at various times in my life and career, and while I have not figured it all out, I want to share a bit about my journey in the hopes that it may provide insight for your own.

Courage as Vulnerability

I come from a strong line of independent women—who learned to change their own tires and their own oil, raised families where crying served no purpose, and quitting was never an option. As a young person growing and watching these women—my mother, my aunts—I learned that where I am from, courage is defined as unfailing perseverance, a constant pursuit of perfection.

A few years ago, my family experienced an incredible tragedy; we lost my brother-in-law to early onset Alzheimer's. He was 37. As you might imagine, this was devastating to my sister and her four children, and our family came together to survive this pain. Over the years that followed, I spent more time than I ever had with my sister. We began to talk about this concept of courage. As we shared our experiences of feeling like our worth was tied to being the best leader or mother, we talked about where it began and wondered whether it still served the value it had when we were kids.

I don't recall how I fell into Brené Brown's work, but it was around this time. And by grace or serendipity, I read her book, *Daring Greatly: How the Courage to Be Vulnerable Transforms the Way We Live, Love, Parent and Lead*. In it, Brown ties the idea of courage or bravery to the concept of vulnerability, which she defines as "showing up and letting ourselves be seen." She goes on to say, "When we spend our lives waiting until we're perfect or bulletproof before we walk into the arena, we ultimately sacrifice relationships and opportunities that may not be recoverable, we squander our precious time, and we turn our backs on our gifts, those unique contributions that only we can make."

Courage as a Decision

If courage is vulnerability and vulnerability is showing up and letting yourself be seen, then the decision to be courageous can start in small ways and at any time. Over the course of your life and career, you will be presented with many opportunities to practice courage. From education, to residency training, to employment, to management and leadership, to building and raising a family (if that is something you choose), and beyond, you will have choices about whether or not to show up and let yourself be seen. *Do you choose to bring your whole self to your workplace? To your mentee or mentoring roles? To your professional organizations?* In my own personal and professional life, I have had many opportunities to choose to be courageous and vulnerable.

Some of the ways we choose to practice courage can be small. For example, I keep the tissues in my office sitting on my desk, in plain view. You might ask, "Why is that courageous?" As a learning manager I was taught that to avoid people crying in your office, one should simply hide the Kleenex. Almost every manager or leader I have worked with has had a box of tissues tucked away somewhere in a cabinet or cupboard, but never prominently displayed.

This strategy to avoid connecting made sense to me. I knew from my own personal experience as a young person that connecting to people could be risky. While attending Alateen, a program to support children living in families with an alcoholic, I learned that the behaviors of alcoholics were not in my control. This was a valuable lesson at this point in my life. However, I internalized this to mean that distancing myself from others offered emotionally protective value, that it was easier to make hard decisions when there was space between myself and others.

Using this tactic in my work life seemed to serve the same emotionally protective mechanism. For example, it allowed me to manage the pain of firing employees I knew to be good human beings when they weren't meeting the expectations of their jobs. It allowed me to distance myself from responding with compassion to a person's tears or sadness and focus solely on correcting employee behavior.

For many, tears are a natural response to stress or even happiness. In the moment when a person is crying, it is easy for the person crying to feel imperfect and to feel shame. It is easy for a person crying to think, "I need to get myself under control." The last thing a person suffering or experiencing shame wants to do is ask for a tissue. A short time ago, not long after my introduction to the concept of vulnerability as courage, I removed the tissue box from the drawer where it had lived for years. I moved it out and displayed it prominently.

This is my simple and subtle attempt at encouraging vulnerability and honoring those who enter my office. It has become a conversation-starter to talk to others about this concept of vulnerability and what it truly means to be supportive, to demonstrate empathy, to say, "This space is a safe space. Cry as much as you want. Here are the tissues." It also serves as a gesture to signal to those entering my office that if they cry, it is OK. This tactic is particularly powerful when I think about how committed I was to avoiding emotional engagement with the people I worked with and the power and strength I have found in connection.

Courage as a Practice

Courage is doing the hard thing. And the hard thing changes over time. Every new opportunity comes with its own set of challenges and potential consequences. If we know that every environment and every decision has the capacity for courage, how can we prepare? Practice, practice, practice.

Think of the first thing you ever did that felt brave. What was it? Riding a scary rollercoaster? Learning how to drive? Choosing to attend college far from home? What does courage look like for you now? Selecting a residency? Caring for an aging parent? Looking for a new job? Parenting a child? What feels courageous may change over our lifetimes, but the need for courage never stops.

Over the course of my career, the hardest thing I have done is make the decision to live my life as an openly lesbian woman. I have lived my life since my mid-twenties committed to talking about my life the way anyone would talk about theirs. When someone asked about my weekend, I made small commitments, like not using vague pronouns and giving my partner's gender. My friends have always known and met people I was dating. Although the courage required to do this has evolved with each new city or job, I only ever shared as much as was necessary to feel normal in any situation. I only let people see as much of me as was necessary to manage my fear.

When I met my wife, she inspired me to speak more freely about being a lesbian, to move from passive acknowledgment to active rejoicing. And so, recently, I have. I share my story with students, with colleagues, and with mentees; I have even shared my story in a nationally published article recently. When I share, I talk about how hard it can be, how it feels like you'll never know when a friend or colleague will step away rather than lean in to learn more, but I also share the joy. The joy of finding bosses and mentors that support you, work environments that are diverse, and those friends and colleagues that celebrate with you. Although I have certainly had some responses encouraging me to share less broadly or to be more quiet about this part of who I am, I have been overwhelmingly encouraged by the responses of many others. I have found that there are many who have a loved one or a friend they want to support and they ask questions about how to do this.

For example, I was asked several years ago to speak to a colleague whose daughter was beginning to identify as gay. I was honored and terrified. I was not close with this colleague, and it was frightening to think of sharing so much of myself. It was also exciting to think that through this sharing of my story, I might impact the future of this mother–daughter relationship in a positive way. We set up an initial call where I shared my story, ideas about what parents can do, and resources for her and her daughter. We connected a few more times. This moment where I showed up and let myself be seen came with great reward. My story helped a mother and her daughter tackle things together, and they have a strong relationship now.

Sometimes, I have found that sharing this part encourages others who have wondered or struggled with the same thing. Frequently, I find this response among students who find me after class or set appointments with me to share and ask questions. Increasingly, schools and colleges of pharmacy are initiating these conversations, inviting leaders to speak openly about what can be done to better honor our students and colleagues for who they are. In these moments, I never miss an opportunity to impart the joy of being honored for all of who you are and the value of honoring all of yourself.

As pharmacists, we will always be faced with tough decisions. Some will be personal, and some will impact patient care. There are moments when we disagree with those we respect because we know a better way. Moments when we know there is a better treatment, better therapy, or simply a better course. There are times when it is important that we speak out in groups, knowing we do not carry the opinion of the majority. Moments that demand a tough decision. *We must show up and let ourselves be seen.*

Brené Brown would say "It's a practice, not an attitude" and that "You can choose courage or you can choose comfort. You cannot choose both." *Choose the hard thing. Be imperfect. Be vulnerable. Be courageous.*

Sincerely,

Lindsey

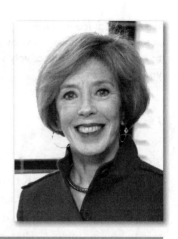

Patricia D. Kroboth
PhD

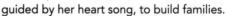

Listening to Your Heart Song While Facing a Challenge

When you spend time with Patricia, it is readily apparent—often within minutes—that you are in the presence of someone who combines a rare mix of extraordinary intelligence, kindness, compassion, humor, a sense of adventure, and a profound ability to nurture. When visitors ask students at the University of Pittsburgh School of Pharmacy about the school's greatest attributes, they routinely mention their access to the dean and her commitment to them. During faculty members' presentations, she is always in the background, with the demeanor of a proud parent, listening and adding supportive comments. When talking about her nieces, nephews, students, or faculty, it is impossible to miss the pride and affection in her eyes. Parental nurturing is a dimension of her being. She infuses her relationships with her biological and professional families with caring that is founded in her commitment to support them as they vigorously pursue their strengths and talents. In her letter, Patricia talks about deeply personal experiences and describes her commitment, guided by her heart song, to build families.

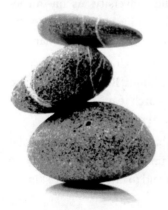

Patricia is currently Dean of the Pittsburgh School of Pharmacy. She is an elected Fellow of the American College of Clinical Pharmacy, the American Association of Pharmaceutical Scientists, and the American Association for the Advancement of Science. She has held elected office in several organizations and is the recipient of the American College of Clinical Pharmacology Bristol Meyers Squibb Mentor Award. She received her BS in Pharmacy from the University at Buffalo SUNY and her MS and PhD (1983) from the University of Pittsburgh.

Patricia's advice is: **Look at your strengths, your talents, and listen to your heart song. We each have a set of personal challenges—often ones that are difficult to share. Dealing effectively with those challenges may lead you to the reason you are here on earth.**

Dear Colleague,

Shortly after I was invited to write you a letter, I saw Oprah on "Good Morning America." I knew instantly that her simple message captured the essence of what I wanted to say. To digress momentarily, my invitation to write a letter was based on thinking that I might share my experiences as a woman in a male-dominated research environment. That is a story for another time. Back to Oprah. As she so eloquently stated when answering a question of a young guest on the show,

> "The highest honor on earth that you will ever have is the honor of being yourself. Your only true job as a human being is to discover why you . . . are here. . . . Every one of us has an internal guidance system, a GPS, an intuition . . . a heart song. Your only job is to listen and discern when it is speaking."

My focus is on something much more personal: my experience with the honor of being myself—and with infertility. I attended graduate school after practicing pharmacy for several years in truly wonderful settings that gave me an amazing set of experiences. Graduate school was a tough decision because I was used to being a financial equal partner with my husband. Once at the University of Pittsburgh, I totally immersed myself in the fabulous opportunities around me. I loved everything about my role—each of them! I went from being a clinician to obtaining my PhD, building a research program, starting the Clinical Pharmaceutical Scientist PhD Program, and building a wonderful team that included students and people internal and external to the University. As my forties approached, I realized my biological clock was truly running out of time. Sadness struck, and the reality that my husband and I would be childless struck hard.

In the meantime, I had developed a work family where fun and laughter were generously interspersed with hard work and long hours. Regular dinners and celebrations at our home, rollerblading with our research team, hiking trips, and more took place with my work family, which included my husband.

In my personal life, our younger sisters were having children. My husband and I prided ourselves on being the best aunt and uncle we could possibly be to each and every one of them. At one point, my mom said to me, "You have skipped being a mother and have become a grandmother."

The oldest of my younger sisters had the first "grandchild" of our families. Soon thereafter, she became a single mom to her son. As he got older, she allowed him to take annual spring vacations with my husband and me, and to stay with us during summers as they lived at a distance. He decorated his room in our home so that it was his room, not our guest room. We were all happy. Then tragedy struck with my sister's diagnosis of multiple myeloma. Sadly, she died at too young an age. Because of our incredible bond with our nephew and our long history of being a second set of parents, our precious young man felt a true part of our little family as he dealt with his loss.

Suddenly, I realized that I had discovered why I was here on this earth. It was crystal clear. I had done my true job as a human being of discovering why I was here. I had unknowingly built an extended biological family where my husband and I were primary in our surrogate son's life. I had also built a work family of students and colleagues. In my heart, I know that I would not have been able to spend the time with them had we had our own children as a young couple.

Today, I have the pleasure of looking back and marveling at the accomplishments of all of my children, who include former students and faculty members who have matured into pharmacists and scientists, senior faculty, and national leaders. It includes our nieces and nephews who have become fine, accomplished young women and men. And, of course, it includes our surrogate son, our nephew. I am not sure what having a biological son would be like. However, I don't think I could love him more. He has grown into a person who people say has characteristics of his biological parents and of my husband and me. As he now starts his own family, I am thrilled that my husband and I will have a special part in his young family.

My message to you is to look at your strengths, your talents, and listen to your heart song. I had two heart songs. My heart song was building the happiest family everywhere I had that opportunity—at work and at home. My heart song was also in my deep-seated passion for my profession and the ways I could contribute. We each have a set of personal challenges—often ones that are difficult to share. Dealing effectively with those challenges may lead you to the reason you are here on earth. I built as many components of our academic program at PittPharmacy that I had the ability to build. Although it was never my intention to be dean, following my heart song brought me to lead our School of Pharmacy. Little did I know that my personal disappointment would eventually allow me to experience such overwhelming joy in both my professional and personal lives. I understand the honor of being myself. And I do believe that I discovered why I am on this earth.

I wish you the very best as you follow your heart song, overcome your personal challenges, and discover why you are on this earth.

With all my best wishes for you,

Patricia

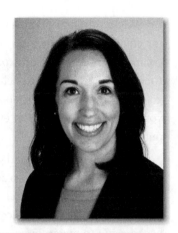

Jennifer Loucks
PharmD, BCPS

Work–Life Balance Is Baloney

Jennifer is a clinical coordinator and new mom who shares her journey in developing a career and personal life. She outlines specific ways she and her husband make their lives work. Her approach focuses on minimizing the guilt about working while also raising a young daughter.

Jennifer is currently Clinical Coordinator–Ambulatory Pharmacy Services and Residency Program Director, postgraduate year 2 (PGY2) ambulatory care pharmacy residency, The University of Kansas Health System, Kansas City, Kansas. Previously she was Clinical Pharmacist–Ambulatory Solid Organ Transplant/Hepatology. She received her PharmD (2009) from The University of Kansas, School of Pharmacy, Lawrence, Kansas and completed an ASHP-accredited PGY1 pharmacy practice residency and PGY2 solid organ transplant/immunology residency at Houston Methodist Hospital, Houston, Texas.

Jennifer's advice is: **Do not look at life as a flat road but rather as peaks and valleys. Trying to achieve a work–life balance is like expecting to only find that flat road.**

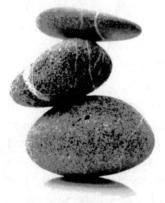

Dear Colleague,

A lot of time is spent talking about work–life balance and how to obtain it. Even more time is spent trying to achieve it. Although it's important to devote time to each, I'm not sure that balance is what we should strive for. I would argue that ***balance is baloney***. I must admit I didn't come up with this concept myself. I attended a talk that focused on this theme, and it has stuck with me.

When you think about a work–life balance, you're usually focused on striving for equilibrium between the two. The statement itself implies that there is a competition between the two: your work and your life are competing for your time. If you are trying to achieve this type of balance, you are almost always going to produce an imbalance resulting in a feeling of failure or guilt. So, ask yourself if it makes sense at every point in our lives to devote equal amounts of ourselves to work and to life. I would argue it does not.

Throughout your life and your career, it makes more sense to tilt the scales in one direction or the other to achieve satisfaction and growth instead of balance. Residency is an example. You are taking one or two years of your life to train to gain the skills and experiences of three to five years in practice. *Do you think you're going to maintain equilibrium between work and life during those years?* No, almost certainly not and that's OK. For many pharmacists, part of the reason they complete a residency is to dedicate time to learn the skills and knowledge necessary to practice in a specific position or obtain their dream job. By taking a year or two and focusing more time on work than life, you can obtain your dream job faster. Then you can shift the equilibrium the other way and focus a bit more on life, while maintaining an enjoyable and rewarding career. Conversely, if you are only focused on maintaining a balance between work and life, and for this reason alone didn't dedicate those years to training, it will probably take you much longer to achieve your dream job. Additionally, you run the risk of being less satisfied with work while on this path. By putting the right amount of your focus on work or life at various times, you can achieve satisfaction in both.

I believe it's entirely possible to love both your work and your non-work lives. Furthermore, work is a huge part of life; so if you don't like your work, figure out what you need to change to start loving it. If you enjoy what you do, work isn't work. Let me tell you a bit of my story.

I truly enjoyed my two years of residency. I was very focused on work and although I developed strong relationships with my co-residents, I was far from maintaining balance or equilibrium between work and life. Much more of my time and energy went to work because it was an opportunity to get everything I could out of those years. During my training years, my shift was toward work and away from life.

After completing my residency, I had my dream job. I was a clinical pharmacist, taking care of patients with the disease state I loved. I had opportunities to complete research, teach, and work with students and residents. All things I had wanted to do. I had job satisfaction. Additionally, I was finally able to focus on life more. I could spend time with friends and family, try new restaurants, work out, cook, travel, and do all the other things I loved to do—*all* because I dedicated myself to work during residency. Even then, I didn't strive for a balance between the two. Because I had satisfaction with both, I didn't mind dedicating extra time to work because I didn't dread work; I really enjoyed it.

Then things changed. My father passed away suddenly, and it was time to tilt the scales again. I lived in Texas, and my newly widowed mother lived in South Dakota and I needed to be there for her. Family comes first, and it was time to focus more on life and less on work. I took a few weeks off, but once I was back at work, I continued to focus on life. I maintained my career, but this was the time to say "no" to an extra research project or presentation. It was time to focus on life, and take care of myself and my family.

As we all know well, life is far from simple or stagnant. Do not look at it as a flat road but rather as peaks and valleys. Trying to achieve a work–life balance is like expecting to only find that flat road. Don't try to do it; *balance is baloney*, and you should focus on work and life in the amount you need at each point in your life. I don't want this message to be misconstrued that you should focus on life so much that you do a poor job at work— that is far from the case. You can absolutely be successful at both. It's important to figure out how to do both well because, as your life and your career grow, you will be depended on more in both. Sometimes this will occur at the same time, sometimes at different times. *The ability to tip your scale in the correct direction at the right time is critical for your overall happiness and success.*

Take, for example, my current situation. My husband and I recently had our first child, who is now 5 months old. I have been back at work for about 2 months, and numerous people have asked me things like: *"How is it being back? Do you wish you were home? Are you glad to be back?"* I have thought a lot about this, and talked to other moms in similar situations. What I keep going back to is the feeling that I want to do both. I'm not sad to go to work, because I enjoy my work. I also love to be with our daughter, so I wish I could do both full time. Both are incredibly important to me, so I've tried to figure out a way to do both while not driving myself crazy or over-extending and doing a poor job at one or the other.

At the same time, my responsibilities at work have grown. I took on a new role as a clinical coordinator and as a Residency Program Director that included starting a new residency program. Just because I was a new mom didn't mean I couldn't continue to advance my career and do things I enjoyed at work to maintain a job that I loved. I had to figure out a way to continue to be dedicated to work while managing my personal life and giving my family enough time. *So how does one do this?*

First, remember, you don't have to be bad at work to be a good parent, and you don't have to be a bad parent to be good at work! You can absolutely be good at both. Also, this doesn't just apply to parenting. It could be anything in your life—a relationship, a hobby, or anything that's important to you.

There are only so many hours in the day, so you need to make every moment count. Always focus on being efficient and effective with your time and actions. What I try to do is plan my day and prioritize tasks at work so that I can leave work each day in time to get home and spend dedicated time with our daughter before she goes to bed. Because this is only a few hours each day, I have also committed to making that time just for her. I'm not on e-mail, doing household chores, or running errands. I can return to those things later in the evening when she is in bed if I need to. ***So how do you do this? There is no easy answer, and I am far from an expert, but here are a few things I've tried that have worked:***

- Take advantage of modern conveniences and technology like online shopping. (I don't know how I survived before Amazon prime!)

- Get organized. Make lists electronically and share them with others they apply to. Then, remember to delegate. Leaders in every field talk about delegating tasks—apply this to your personal life as well as at work.

- Hire someone to do your household chores that take your valuable time. As an example, I use a cleaning service.

- Plan a menu, use grocery delivery, and prepare meals/ingredients ahead. This is one of my most important steps. Don't feel guilty for sending your children to day care. Think about how they benefit from being there.

- Try to avoid expending energy on trivial issues. Have perspective instead of stressing or stewing over things. If you need to address a situation, figure out a plan and address it. Otherwise, let it go.

- Schedule time for yourself; don't forget this. It helps to keep you sane.

- Follow the 1-minute rule. If it's takes less than 1 minute to do something, just do it when it comes up and don't put it off.

Finally, remember, you can't force a timeline. We all have an idea in our heads of when things should happen in our lives and professional careers, but this is only a starting point. Life will throw you curves, and you need to adapt to them. Keep an open mind and lean on others around you. I didn't invent any of these ideas on my own. Like pharmacy students and residents observing numerous pharmacists to develop their own practice, I have learned these things from talking to lots of people and implementing what works for me. Continue to evaluate your focus on work and life and make sure you are putting the right amount of time into each to achieve your goals. If you aren't where you want to be in either your life or your career, don't feel like you can't get there. You aren't limited to getting all of this done in a certain way or during a certain window of time. Think about what is lacking and how you can focus on one or the other—or both—to achieve success and satisfaction.

Balance is baloney, so focus on what makes sense at each point in your life and you can have both a job and a life that you love. Life is short; make the most of it!

Sincerely,

Jenny

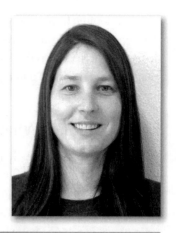

Ellen Maddox
PharmD, BCPS

Growing from Adversity

Ellen shares her experiences in striving toward her goals and what *not* reaching some have taught her, including lessons that resulted from a divorce and becoming a single parent. She includes how she has progressed from a little *I* leader to a big *L* leader.

Ellen is currently Clinical Coordinator, Legacy Health System Salmon Creek Medical Center, in Vancouver, Washington, where previously she was a clinical staff pharmacist. She received her PharmD (2010) from the University of Washington School of Pharmacy, Seattle, Washington. She completed an ASHP-accredited postgraduate year (PGY) 1 pharmacy practice residency at Peace Health Southwest Medical Center, in Vancouver, Washington.

Ellen's advice is: I realize that no matter how much stability we desire, there will always be chaos (big or small) and change to overcome. Becoming a leader requires you to work through challenges and be confident that you can overcome the obstacles you might face in the present and in the future.

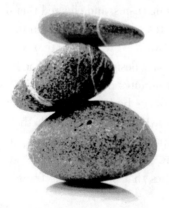

Dear Colleague,

If you had asked me 15 years ago to give an example of a leader, I would have probably mentioned a formal leader, such as an organization's chief executive officer or a political figure. If there is one thing I have learned since that time, it is the realization that leadership can take on many forms. I am a female, former collegiate athlete, young practitioner, divorced single parent—and I have become a leader in my profession as a pharmacist.

Developing into a leader has been a progressive process—one that has developed over time and through personal experiences. I have found the greatest areas of growth occurred not only in times of success, but also during periods of change and hardship. I'd like to share with you some of the lessons learned that have shaped my journey to becoming a leader.

Understanding What It Means to Be a Leader

It may surprise you that my path to leadership began with athletics. Becoming a pharmacist and playing collegiate basketball were both goals that I had set for myself early on. I was fortunate to be recruited by a college that provided me the opportunity to pursue both. During my junior year, my team had a breakout year after a coaching change propelled my team to a 28-7 record and a National Association of Intercollegiate Athletics (NAIA) championship berth—the first in school history. The following season, I continued to get some quality minutes coming off the bench. My strength was my defensive presence, and I accepted the role in pushing my teammates to improve. As a team, we weren't a group of all-stars but prided ourselves on execution and hard work in the gym and class-room; it was physically and mentally demanding. We worked together, regardless of how many minutes we played, toward the same goal—winning. Unfortunately for me, about midway through the season, I never made it back on to the court. I didn't have an injury, a bad attitude, or off-court issues; my coach just simply didn't give me the opportunity to play. Despite this decision, I still approached every weight-lifting session, film review, and practice with a positive attitude. I found myself having to mask my disappointment, anger, and sadness over the end of my collegiate career.

I still struggle with the decision my coach made that year, but appreciate that this experience brought about personal growth. My teammates would say I helped them become better players through my hard work and perseverance. I pushed them to improve, prepped them for opposing teams, and cheered them on from the sidelines. At the end of the year, the team captains presented me with an award they deemed "The True Teammate Award." It was a title that was uncomfortable for me at that time, but I now see it as a designation for a leader. Ultimately, it wasn't a matter of playing the most minutes or being the team's leading scorer. It was earning my teammates' respect by demonstrating the development of early leadership characteristics: growth in individual skills that supported the team, the tenacity to work hard, coping with setbacks, making a commitment and following through, managing my emotions, and focusing on achieving our team goal. It was these characteristics that provided the frame-work for my leadership growth.

Learning to Be a Leader

After college, I began pharmacy school and started an internship at a local hospital that unexpectedly became my springboard for learning about leadership within the pharmacy profession. My mentors had designed a program to specifically develop young leaders and facilitate opportunities to gain leadership experience. My mentors stressed the importance of being a leader. I expanded my knowledge about leadership through focused studies, hands-on projects, one-on-one mentoring, and discussions about challenges of leadership in the "real-world." This guidance inspired me to seek out more formal roles of leadership in the academic setting and within national organizations. I also consciously took on an expanded role among my peers in the workplace. I built on the leadership qualities I had gained through athletics and incorporated them into a new setting. I gained confidence in my ability to lead, on a small scale, and gained new skills in organization, communication, and conflict resolution.

At the time, I didn't fully appreciate the impact that the direct and indirect teaching moments with my mentors would have in my next steps as a leader. During my residency and the years to follow, I used the concepts of lean, emotional intelligence, little "L" leaders to develop my leadership skills. I found mentors who shared their knowledge, provided constructive feedback, and challenged me to engage in leadership opportunities. *During this time, I learned several lessons:*

- The importance of *identifying and working with a strong mentor*. My mentors throughout my personal and professional life provided stability and guidance. They shared knowledge and experiences as well as encouraged me to pursue a leadership path.

- My leadership growth could not have progressed without learning the attributes of a leader. I became a "student of leadership" whenever possible. This knowledge was gained through *studying leadership concepts* and listening and learning from my mentors and peers.

- *Practicing leadership whenever possible*. I took advantage of opportunities to develop, exercise, and build a leadership skillset. Application of leadership concepts into real situations helped me learn from my mistakes and successes. The more I was able to lead a group or take on an expanded role within my team, the more I was able to define myself as a leader.

Becoming a Leader

About five years ago, I was ready for a change and left the organization where I had worked during and following residency. In my new position, I focused on opportunities for leadership, taking the lead on precepting rotations, assisting with electronic medical record (EMR) enhancements, and participating in longitudinal projects at a site and system level. Along with many positive changes in my professional career, came some big changes in my personal life: buying my first home, becoming a mother, and coping with an emotionally abusive relationship.

This year, I found myself having to navigate through a divorce, sell my home, take on a large financial burden, and also become a single parent. Despite my best efforts, my personal challenges significantly impacted my day-to-day life. It also added to the stress of meeting on-the-job responsibilities, maintaining an active role in my ongoing projects, and working a variable schedule. I maintained a positive attitude, but I also found it difficult to share with co-workers the hardships I was facing. My athletic experiences had prepared me well for coping with adversity, and my former teammates were the people I turned to for guidance. They kept me focused while I worked through those hard times. I used my skills to cope, while handling my emotions and putting forth my best efforts at work. They kept in close contact, provided basic necessities (clothes, a car, housing), helped with childcare, etc. They also reminded me that I deserved the best and made me realize that I had worked hard to achieve recognition in my profession. That year, a pharmacy clinical coordinator position at my organization became available. It was a position that I considered my dream job; however, I initially hesitated to apply because it didn't feel like the right time. I was just beginning to settle my personal affairs and felt comfortable in my current position. As a relatively new practitioner, I doubted I was ready to step into a formal management role. *Would I be able to balance the stressors of a new position with my personal life? Did being a female and single parent affect my chances? Would I be able to meet my co-workers' and department's expectations?*

I spent the next month reflecting on how I would balance a new leadership role. I recognized that it would be challenging if I didn't make adjustments to my personal life: setting a daily routine, adopting a meal-planning program, and dedicating specific time for family (daily/weekly). Lastly, I started asking for help from others. I sought out a counselor to talk through the past year's challenges, met with friends regularly, and asked friends and family for childcare assistance. I leaned on co-workers for support in managing at-work stressors. They became my leadership mentors (personally and professionally). Ultimately, it took small changes in thinking positively, managing my time, and asking for support to become a happier person, mother, and professional. It enabled me to find a successful balance in my work and home life to feel more confident to pursue a new role. During the interview process, I sometimes felt like the prior year's personal events overshadowed my qualities as a leader. I feared my past personal relationship that had held me back would continue to keep me from moving forward.

Finally, pursuing and ultimately becoming a formal leader was not what I had expected. The opportunity arose when I least expected it; for many reasons, it felt like it was not the right time to pursue a change in my career. It would have been easy to pass up the opportunity, continue in my comfort zone, or wait until the timing felt right. However, I was reminded of my personal growth to leadership and how my experiences had prepared me to take on the new role. I realized that no matter how much stability we desire, there will always be chaos (big or small) and change to overcome. Becoming a leader requires you to work through challenges and be confident that you can overcome the obstacles you might face in the present and in the future.

Cultivating Leadership

Each phase or chapter of my life has helped me grow into the leader that I am today. ***During these phases, there are several common elements:***

- ***People.*** Surround yourself with people who will support you. My teammates, mentors, family, friends, and co-workers listened, questioned, and encouraged me in my journey personally and professionally. They saw me through times of grief and times of great success. The people you engage with are an essential element to shaping the type of leader you will become.

- ***Vision.*** Have a goal in mind. Whether you are chasing a conference championship, an advanced degree, or a promotion, make sure to know what the end goal is and the steps to get there. Find ways to move forward.

- ***Balance.*** In times of stability or change, it can be difficult to find the right combination of input versus output. Being efficient, fueling yourself (through learning, hard work, reflection), and not stressing about things out of your control will help balance the external factors that affect your day-to-day decisions as a leader.

- ***Confidence.*** Lack of skills or experience should never hold you back. Be confident in what role you play on your team, in learning, and in challenging yourself to do new things. If you prepare well and have the passion to do something, you should be confident in what you have to offer as a leader.

As I embrace my new role as a formal leader, I will continue to reflect on my past lessons, achievements, and goals as I strengthen my skills. I hope that regardless of your leadership phase, you will recognize that you, too, can become a leader.

All the best,

Ellen

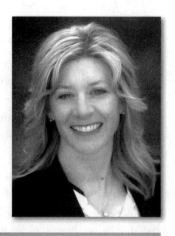

Julie R. McCoy
PharmD

Amid Life's Challenges, Hold True to Your Values

Julie is a busy pharmacist with several "irons in the fire" who is grateful for life's gifts. Julie is a pharmacy leader, a mom of four, and a law student.

Julie is currently Assistant Director of Pharmacy, Quality and Medication Safety and Director, postgraduate year 1 (PGY1) pharmacy residency program, Pharmacy Services, Providence SW Washington Region, Olympia, Washington, and Clinical Professor, Adjunct Faculty, Washington State University, College of Pharmacy. Julie is also an Affiliate Faculty member, University of Washington, School of Pharmacy. Julie received her BS in Pharmacy and PharmD (1997) at Washington State University and is currently completing her law degree at Mitchell Hamline School of Law, with an anticipated graduation in 2019.

Julie's advice is: **Plan for your success, hold true to your values, support those who are less fortunate, practice gratitude, celebrate your achievements, and smile as often as possible.**

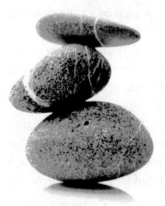

Dear Colleague,

My journey has been about holding true to my values despite life's challenges. Although some of my toughest battles have been related to being a woman, wife, and mom, I have learned to overcome challenges by making each success about being a better person. In addition, in raising three boys, I find strength in allowing them to learn by observing my imperfections, because they know my bar is very high. They also understand that I will hold them accountable for their own kindness, respect, and integrity. Living through challenging situations has forced me to self-reflect and learn more about what is most important to me; here I will share a few insights with you.

First, I find value in sponsoring the underdog and spending the extra time and energy to support those with special needs. I am a second child in a family of four children, but I became the surrogate oldest sibling because my older brother was born with a developmental disability. Despite being ridiculed and teased by youth who did not understand how to react to his disability, he carved out his own mainstream and endured. He found joy in the simple things in life, standing in my doorway before bedtime, telling me about his day, and asking for my opinion about life's questions as I drifted off to sleep. He practiced football and other sports with his teammates, but saw very little playing time; still he enjoyed reveling as a champion on championship teams. During high school graduation, he received a standing ovation when he was awarded the certificate for having missed only one day during all of high school. His surprise and beaming smile in his emotional acceptance of the award demonstrated his sense of accomplishment and pride in his education.

While I focused on my goal of becoming a pharmacist, my brother celebrated the successes of the Seattle Seahawks and the Seattle Super Sonics, or he was surly for their losses; he always created a good laugh and a break from the intensity level that I imposed on myself. I spoke up for his well-being on more than one occasion, and the principal of the school definitely knew my name. Families are not perfect. Life isn't always fair. My journey with my brother taught me to advocate for those who are not as well-equipped, to enjoy the simple pleasures in life, and to treasure time with those you love.

Second, as I look back at pharmacy school, I realize how influential my teachers were, and how important it is to plan for lifelong connections. The most memorable professors in pharmacy school were individuals who stopped to write a letter of recommendation for me or who advocated for life-changing research projects that ultimately changed the trajectory of my career. Professors and mentors who led by example and who I held in high regard are now collaborating with teams at Centers for Medicare & Medicaid Services (CMS), working as pharmacy executives across multiple states, and even working as pharmacy executives in Switzerland and Wales. They deserved respect then, and they are even more highly regarded now. When I reach out to them even years later, they still reach back. In pharmacy school, my career was only just getting started so I was unable to envision my professional future. Now I know how much time it takes to teach, and I appreciate the time they invested in me as a student. My point here is to realize you may come across your teachers and mentors again, so treat them with respect and learn everything you can from them. As we become mentors, the same concept applies for our own students—use the gift of influence wisely.

Third, find your own work productivity and pace, as it relates to your future vision. Like most pharmacists, I prefer to be on the edge of crazy-busy most days, with just enough time to grab a snack and a quick walk. I enjoy accomplishing more and more each year, and I prefer to keep as many doors open as possible. After residency, I practiced first as an emergency department clinical pharmacist, and then moved into leadership roles involving quality, safety, and pharmacy residency. As I embraced leadership and spent less time in clinical practice, I had to make decisions about which direction my career would go. Although being a pharmacist offers almost endless professional opportunities, I had an inner drive to find the intersection where healthcare and legal risk or benefit come together.

My friends and family asked why I would be interested in law school when I have been blessed with such an interesting and rewarding career as a pharmacist. It's simple. I enjoy my work each and every day, and my hope is that this law degree will make my future career even more interesting when combined with the foundational pharmacy backdrop. Wouldn't it be exciting to work with the Food and Drug Administration (FDA), CMS, industry, the Joint Commission, or with healthcare providers—always with patients as the focus? Statistics show I may need to work for many years to come, and law is a new and exciting language that I am just beginning to speak. I love being a pharmacist, but I feel that something greater is out there. That is what drove me to pursue a law degree.

In my law school program, students complete coursework in a hybrid model over roughly four years, spending at least 51% of their time face-to-face, with the remainder on-line. The meaning of *evidence-based practice* is different in law school than in medicine, as legal precedent can come from many sources (federal, state, case law) and paradigm cases can be from long ago but still represent good law. Therefore, the reading must be completed with deliberate intent to understand the material. Subjects like criminal law were foreign to me and required extra time. I learned the importance of using "Lean" strategies to become as organized as possible, and I found that there are creative ways to capture minutes of the day. The majority of my days begin at 4:00 a.m., and I am out of the office at least one week per semester to attend capstone week in Minnesota. I am thankful for the support from leaders at my hospital, including my pharmacy director. I learned that it is indeed possible to work full time and complete law school. My recommendation here is to keep learning, pursue life planning, for both professional and personal life choices, so that you always have your own vision and pace in mind. ***Reflect, take a deep breath, stay true to your goals, and use your time wisely.***

Finally, one of the biggest challenges in my journey has been how to handle dust, dishes, laundry, and life's surprises during a busy day or week. I chose to be a pharmacist, and I cherish my career. I wouldn't trade my children for anything. I value the partnership with my husband. We have a dog, two goats, and three chickens, and they all need food and water. Everybody needs something. While I was in law school, my family welcomed a baby girl. After having three boys, we were presented with a delightful gift! She could not be planned for, and the timing ended up being fantastic because it takes a small village to raise her. Who knew teenage boys would be so entertained by their sister giving them the "evil eye," while throwing food under her highchair to the dog Ashley waiting anxiously below? Then they all laugh while Ashley cleans the floor. They encourage each other and they are drawn to each other, bringing us all closer as a family.

Each of our boys visited the emergency department in the last year, and luckily the result was only two broken bones and a few missed sporting events. Each time, we learned to put everything else aside as we were reminded to be thankful for good health and excellent healthcare providers. We learned to become more efficient with our time, share in responsibilities, and shop online when possible. My husband has stepped up to do the lion's share of cooking and cleaning, and I'm more than OK with that. We joke that he is mister safe and mister clean—a definite reflection of his extremely satisfying career choice as a firefighter–paramedic. Thank goodness we also have three sets of grandparents to help and keep us grounded. *What's important to me?* Being present, expressing gratitude, and finding joy in knowing that the 15-year-old learns independence through making his own lunch and cleaning the mud off his baseball cleats. When they need me, I'll be there. Solid decisions come with careful thought, intention, and purpose, with flexibility and the understanding that some things simply cannot be scheduled, organized, or calculated according to your expectations.

For me, the journey has been about learning to be a stronger person through the process of overcoming challenges and looking back to understand the lessons meant to be learned. I realize that my lessons are often due to serendipitous conversations with individuals who were facing a challenge on their journey as well. For example, the ASHP Visiting Leaders Program allowed me to discuss personal and professional life planning with inspiring individuals who have experienced what I can only imagine to be rich lives. I have benefited immensely from attempting to incorporate the wisdom of physician and nurse leaders and other spiritual and ethical leaders into my own life choices. *In your journey, I challenge you to plan for your success, hold true to your values, support those who are less fortunate, practice gratitude, celebrate your achievements, and smile as often as possible.*

Sincerely,

Julie

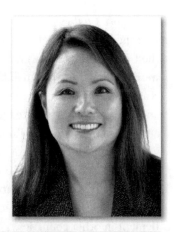

Yen T. Pham
BS Pharm, MBA

Be Persistent and Leave a Footprint

Yen has a unique story to tell, starting with her incredible journey from Vietnam as a child to currently serving in a prominent leadership role in the profession of pharmacy.

Yen is Associate Vice President, Pharmacy Services and Clinical Dietitians, Oregon Health Sciences University Hospital and Clinics, Portland, Oregon. Yen received her BS in Biology and BS in Pharmacy (1997) at the University of Houston. She also completed her MBA in Healthcare Management at the Oregon Health Sciences University (OHSU) School of Medicine, Division of Management.

Yen's advice is: **Leave behind a memorable footprint. You can have confidence that you are a great leader when your team functions at a higher level in your absence!**

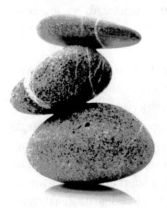

Dear Colleague,

My story is not as typical as other pharmacy leaders. I have not taken a traditional approach to building my career in pharmacy leadership. The journey was not impossible, but it was also not easy. I faced many challenges, opposition, cynicism, and roadblocks. These obstacles never deterred me from my goals and priorities. As such, the challenges helped to build my character, confidence, and the strength I needed for the next level.

Before I tell you my story, let me go back to the beginning. At the age of six, I escaped Vietnam by boat with my father and seven siblings to seek freedom in the United States. We were known as "boat people" or Vietnamese refugees. We were crammed into a small boat with a few hundred other refugees. Food was scarce, and we were provided only bread and water. The ocean journey was long and treacherous. We drifted for three days and two nights before we discovered a small island known as Tarempa, Indonesia. The living conditions in Tarempa were less than ideal. Lack of clean water and poor sanitation resulted in sickness and death among many of our people. After six months, we were evacuated to Galang, Indonesia, in order to avoid a life-threatening tropical typhoon. Galang was considered a temporary safe haven before refugees were processed for resettlement in other countries.

Our family of nine waited for a year and a half to enter the United States. I truly believe this early experience established my core foundation and sustains me now throughout my work and leadership. These adversities taught me the value of being persistent and created a strong determination to prosper. I am reminded of a quote from Jim Watkins: "*A river cuts through rock not because of its power but because of its persistence.*" In fact, possessing this critical trait has propelled me to seek opportunities and find successes throughout my career.

I took a nontraditional route toward a leadership role in pharmacy. After receiving a BS in Pharmacy, I worked as a staff pharmacist in outpatient retail pharmacy. I was promoted to Manager shortly afterward. A year later, I was offered an opportunity to manage a small, family-owned specialty pharmacy. Venturing into specialty pharmacy was my ultimate defining moment and a milestone to jumpstarting my career to pharmacy leadership. Similar to other small, family-owned pharmacies, the pharmacy merged with a larger specialty pharmacy corporation. My curiosity motivated me to learn everything about specialty pharmacy from operations to billing and the complexities of compliance. I credit my success today because of these experiences. After a few years, I found another opportunity and took a position as Pharmacy District Manager for a large retail pharmacy chain.

During my tenure at this company, I was very fortunate to have an excellent manager. She was a great mentor, supportive of me and my career, and a thoughtful leader. I admired her perseverance and work ethic. She had a talent to see the best in people and develop their skills. My approach and leadership styles are patterned after hers. I learned to take a proactive approach in everything I set out to do. Although my accomplishments and leadership skills put me on the list to be the next Regional Vice President, I was at a point in my career where I needed and wanted to learn different things as well as welcome new challenges.

This position allowed me to hone my abilities in all aspects of operations. With the direct or indirect oversight of approximately 200 employees, I have become a more effective pharmacy leader. I managed finances for the department including payroll, operating expenses, and inventory control. By consistently achieving budget and operating goals, I have generated $8 million in sales and revenue. Additionally, I implemented the first urgent care clinic in Oregon to enhance revenue, improve access to care, and lower overall patient costs. In the next stage of my career, I accepted the new position of Assistant Director for Outpatient and Ambulatory Pharmacy Services with OHSU Health System. The wide expanse of interdisciplinary teams taught me how to manage and communicate more effectively.

Since then I have been promoted to Associate Vice President for Pharmacy Services and Clinical Dieticians. During this time, I have devised and implemented key initiatives including home infusion, specialty pharmacy, mail order pharmacy, compounding pharmacy, and pharmacy benefit management services. Additionally, specialty pharmacy has successfully achieved Utilization Review Accreditation Commission (URAC) accreditation. I am accountable for the efficient operation of the ambulatory, clinical, and inpatient pharmacies as well as clinical dietitians, which includes the operations and strategic planning of seven retail outlets, seven infusion pharmacies, a compounding pharmacy, inpatient clinical and distributive services, and research pharmacy services. My responsibilities include establishing standards of quality, productivity, and performance in accordance with the vision, value, and mission of the hospital's policies and procedures and requirements of state and federal regulatory agencies.

My career path from Assistant Director to Associate Vice President has tested my reserve. Earlier on at OHSU, I did not receive a promotion to Director of Pharmacy because I was told I was not qualified for the job. I dealt with ongoing challenges and barriers, including lack of support from key stakeholders. Preconceived ideas of my capabilities have never stood in the way of my success. I respond to this by exhibiting confidence and resoluteness in an environment of doubt. I am not rigid in my thinking and always come prepared with different plans to overcome barriers. My mindset is grounded in solution-oriented thinking, and I tend to see barriers as opportunities for novel solutions. The rejection made me stronger and a better leader. I often remind myself that we learn from failures and rejections—a key component of success and leadership. My goal is always to set a good example for my team members who observe and learn from my actions and decisions. Anticipating and managing roadblocks helps me create successful strategies to drive change. My approach is to continue to do my job well despite the setbacks.

I have been at different levels of pharmacy leadership for over 20 years. I have achieved many successes and failures and have leveraged them as stepping stones to better myself personally and professionally. *Here is my advice and lessons learned for women in leadership:*

- *Be persistent, strong, and always better yourself.* You will face rejections and disappointments. I have had multiple setbacks throughout my career. However, I didn't allow it to deter me from my goals and priorities. I continued on and learned from them.

- *Surround yourself with a team that has different thoughts and ideas.* I have 21 managers with diverse educational experiences and backgrounds. They continue to challenge me. I don't often make the final decision. Most decisions are agreed upon by a majority. This collaborative environment makes it acceptable to have a difference of opinion because we think differently and come up with better ideas. For example, if there is a problem, we convene a meeting to discuss it. I listen to my managers' explanations of the pros and cons to a potential solution. Then, we build on each other's ideas and come up with possible solutions and decide through a vote. Managers appreciate this process because their concerns and ideas are raised and heard. Your team is an extension of you and your leadership. Nurture them and take care of them.

- *Don't rush for the next title.* The knowledge and experiences I have achieved with each position are invaluable. Each one has prepared me to be ready for the next level. If you don't learn from your own failures and successes, then you are not paying attention.

- *Think outside the box by remaining nimble and flexible.* Healthcare is changing constantly. Be ready for the changes and adapt. Your team needs a leader to be ready for sudden changes.

- *Work–life balance is key.* Dedication to your home life is as important as your career. Companies and corporations will move on and thrive with or without you. At the end of day, time with your family is what matters.

- *Always remain calm and cool under pressure.* It is human nature/behavior to label a person, especially a woman, as "irrational" if you show stress or distress under pressure. At this point, people around you will stop listening. Learn how to control and manage your distress/stress. During a tumultuous time, our pharmacy operations were in complete disarray, and I was under a tremendous amount of stress and pressure from senior leadership. Regardless, I stayed in control and worked with my team to strategize and respond to the issues. The result was that I garnered more respect and loyalty from my team.

- *Be loyal to your profession.* People often mistook my dedication and passion as dedication to the companies and/or corporations. As a matter of fact, my dedication centered on my pharmacy profession regardless of my employer. I am truly dedicated and passionate about elevating the pharmacy profession and making it better. My vision includes our pharmacists and technicians practicing at the broadest scope of their licenses, thereby elevating our pharmacy profession to the next level.

- *Manage your boss.* Establish a trusting relationship with your boss. This is critical and can be difficult and challenging. If you can't establish a trusting relationship with your boss after multiple attempts, it is time to move on. Think like your boss and always try to be ten steps ahead of him or her. In order to stay ahead, I have an open-door policy. My team readily shares any relevant information that would affect operations. As such, I relate to my boss the potential issues as well as solutions. Your role is to make your boss shine at the right moment and in the right environment.

- *And lastly...have fun.* Have fun doing your job. I love my job and what I have accomplished. I enjoy the innovations, successes, laughter, and even failures along the way.

As I've taken a quick glance back over my career, I am proud of what I have accomplished. I will continue to expand our footprint to create opportunities for our pharmacy team. I push to elevate and move our pharmacy profession to the next level.

In retrospect, I have to admit that my career path was rough and unstable at times. However, I have no regrets because I have accumulated a lifetime of knowledge along the way and continue to enjoy the journey.

Sincerely,

Yen

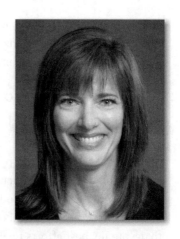

Beth Phillips
PharmD, FCCP, FASHP, BCPS, BCACP

Make Everything Count!

Beth's life is full with professional, family, and personal responsibilities, which she manages by staying organized and passionate about the pharmacy profession.

Beth is currently Rite Aid Professor, Clinical and Administrative Pharmacy, University of Georgia, College of Pharmacy. Beth received her PharmD (1994) at the University of Kansas and completed a pharmacy practice residency at the University of Illinois, Chicago and her ambulatory care specialty residency at the VA Medical Center, Iowa City, Iowa.

Beth's advice is: As you navigate your career, make everything count, pursue your passions and take advantage of opportunities, balance your work and personal lives, and stay organized to meet your professional and personal goals.

Dear Colleague,

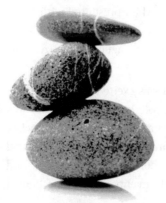

People often ask me, "*How do you do it?*" What they are really asking is how someone balances her responsibilities at work and at home. As I reflect on my career, I realize I have my own story of successes and challenges. What I share is my story; I hope that pieces of it are inspiring and useful in your own career and quest for balance.

Organization is one of my keys to success. It helps me to explain larger ideas or tackle challenges after summarizing the main steps in the path to success or to the solution. To that end, here is a list of what I consider to be the fundamental elements to my success: (1) make everything count, (2) pursue your passions, (3) maintain balance, and (4) stay organized.

Make Everything Count

One of the strategies that I live by in my professional life and gives me balance in my personal life is to make everything count. To me, this means that all of my professional pursuits and opportunities align with my job responsibilities and expectations. As a clinical faculty member, I wear many hats: clinical pharmacist, teacher, and preceptor to students and residents, residency director, researcher, editor, and let's not forget about actively participating in the profession! Trying to devote my best efforts to all of these areas can be challenging. With my daily responsibilities, projects, scholarship, and professional organization involvement, I am always looking for ways to re-tool my work and use it for another purpose. For example, clinical controversies in patient care become topics for research projects, presentations, or review articles. The work dedicated to these efforts in turn enhances the care I provide to patients, and creates good teaching points for students and residents. The professional activities also filter down to patient care and teaching. When I work on a big project, I always find multiple uses for the knowledge gained or work spent by pursuing a professional presentation or peer-reviewed publication. Knowing my professional goals helps me determine what opportunities I should pursue and which ones are not the best fit. It also helps to maintain balance in my personal life because I know which opportunities do not align with my career goals and/or job responsibilities.

Pursue Your Passions

Another guiding principle is to pursue my passions. I am grateful to work in a profession I love that has so many opportunities to get involved and give back. However, it can be difficult to choose or say "no" when presented with these opportunities. For me, I feel deeply committed to residency training. I always said *"yes"* to anything residency-related. Over time, colleagues recognized this and more opportunities followed.

After completing my two years of residency, I was excited to start my first "real" position in the profession. The pharmacist role in ambulatory care was not as robust and widespread as it is today, so we had to establish pharmacists as essential members of the healthcare team. I practiced in primary care and specialty clinics in an academic medical center, where my co-pharmacist and I worked diligently to develop services that would eventually become known as collaborative practice agreements, as well as billing for our services. Luckily, my institution was progressive and suggested that we start an ambulatory care residency. Well, they didn't have to ask me twice—I jumped at the chance! That's when ambulatory care really took off at our institution. The physicians asked for more pharmacy services, and the numbers of pharmacists grew along with services and patient care.

I welcomed the opportunity to direct the residency program and learned as much as possible about the best practices in residency training. I wasn't really sure what to expect for my first residency accreditation survey, and I had more questions about how to improve the program and consequently, advance the profession. I looked to the professional organizations and started networking with others involved in residency training.

Eventually, I was invited to serve as a practitioner surveyor on accreditation survey teams, and later to join the Residency Learning System (now called Residency Program Design and Conduct) faculty and teach in the workshops at professional meetings. I received an opportunity to serve on the ASHP Commission on Credentialing, the body that oversees residency accreditation and develops policies for residency design and conduct. Although the time commitment was considerable (this group is known as one of the hardest working within the organization) in terms of outside work required and time away from my family, I wanted to find a way to fit it all in.

Maintain Balance

Balancing work, family, and personal life can seem like an impossible task at times, and this is one of the universal challenges I see in pharmacists who are entering the profession. They have spent significant amounts of time studying and training in patient care and have had little time for themselves in between all of the other deadlines and projects.

In my case, I chose to start a family a few years after beginning my career. This was ideal for me because I had time to establish myself within the profession and gain confidence in my work and contributions. Colleagues and those in leadership roles routinely called on me to contribute to patient care issues, professional education, and collaboration on research projects, so I felt confident those opportunities would continue to present themselves even if I needed to slow down or temporarily put them on hold. I remember hearing a well-known female pharmacist at a professional meeting explaining that sometimes your professional life takes priority and sometimes your personal life takes priority. I don't think she was the first person to voice this idea, but her words resonated within me. For the first year after each of my two daughters were born, I took some time off and did not seek out as many opportunities for professional contribution. I had worked hard prior to that point and was able to "ride" on some of the publications and outcomes of my previous work. Still, I became more selective in the opportunities I accepted during that time. I needed time to adjust to my new life and develop strategies for organization and getting work done while still providing everything I wanted and needed to do as a mother.

Once I had fully adjusted, I was ready to jump back in and take on more professional involvement. Since then, I found that I adjusted to new efficiencies, such as getting work done at home or during travel downtime, which is something I had not previously considered. Sometimes I need to arrange my personal life to accommodate work deadlines or arrange my work schedule and deadlines to accommodate my family's needs. The key to balancing work responsibilities is collaborating with your colleagues to ensure patients' and learners' needs are met.

Everyone needs some kind of support network to be successful. Some people have a large family network of support. In my case, my parents were older and passed away fairly early on in my career, and my husband's family lives in a different country. My support network for balancing work and family is my husband. He also has a successful career, and we are constantly supporting each other and our family. Although my husband and I are both pharmacists by education, we each have our separate areas of expertise and rarely discuss work at home. We function effectively because we understand the demands of the profession, and it seems we innately know how to balance work and family needs. We share the responsibilities and joys of raising our children, including pick-ups, homework time, meals, and spectating youth sports. This takes constant organization and "calendar management." We have access to a shared calendar so that we aren't scheduled to be out of town on a speaking engagement or residency accreditation survey at the same time. We also have a great network of afterschool nannies—young women who are excellent role models and enjoy spending time with our children.

People often ask me how I find time for myself. To be honest, this can be tough. When you make a choice for your family and your career, these things often come first—and I wouldn't have it any other way. It means that you make time for the important things in life. For me, it means taking trips or a hike with my family, getting together with good friends, and making time to stay in shape. I appreciate the small things such as watching my daughters compete in their respective sports, or having dinner or going for coffee with a colleague or friend when your family members miraculously all have an engagement at the same time. I am also grateful for the "me" time and satisfaction of contributing to society that the profession provides. These things are all possible because I schedule them into my calendar, and work to ensure a good plan for all of my other responsibilities.

Stay Organized

None of my accomplishments would have been possible without staying organized, being on top of deadlines, budgeting time, and getting back to people in a timely manner. This is one of the most important factors to my success. I keep two lists of deadlines at any given time—one is a daily "To Do" list with emails, meetings, or other projects that must be completed that day, and the second is a list of projects such as manuscripts, teaching materials, slide presentations, manuscript reviews, committee work, and other projects with long-term deadlines. I like to use my calendar because it is accessible on my desktop, laptop, and phone. I set reminders for important deadlines, even for small things such as an alert to respond to an email as well as larger commitments like submitting a manuscript. This is my backup in case I get focused on my other deadlines and forget about something I need to do. I especially like having access to my calendar from my phone because I can make notes wherever I am and even when I am not close to my desktop. Being organized means keeping your calendar up-to-date with important work and personal life events so that you can identify a conflict with a particular obligation months in advance.

As you navigate your career, I wish you the best in making everything count, pursuing your passions and taking advantage of opportunities, balancing your work and personal lives, and staying organized to meet all of your professional and personal goals.

All the best,

Beth

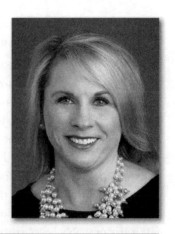

Regina Schomberg
PharmD, BCPS

You Can Have It All, Just Not All at Once

Regina is a midcareer pharmacist who has taken advantage of opportunities by seizing them. She began her practice as a distributive staff pharmacist and moved into clinical practice (nephrology, solid organ, and internal medicine), then on to clinical leadership, and recently transitioned to community and specialty pharmacy.

Regina is currently Assistant Director of Specialty Pharmacy Services and Residency Program Director (RPD), postgraduate year 1 (PGY1) community-based pharmacy residency program, Wake Forest Baptist Health, Winston-Salem, North Carolina. Previously she served as Pharmacy Systems Manager, Community and Specialty Pharmacy, and Residency Program Coordinator, PGY1 pharmacy practice residency program. Regina received her BS (1992) and PharmD (1998) from the University of North Carolina School of Pharmacy, Chapel Hill.

Regina's advice is: Schedule happiness in your day and find that balance between professional obligation and development. Organization is key to having it all.

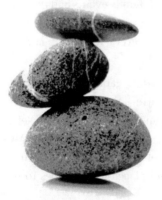

Dear Colleague,

Throughout my life, I have been fortunate to watch women excel at home and in the workplace. These women have mentored me and provided a unique perspective that I am now sharing with young pharmacy professionals. I constantly receive questions such as *"How can I have it all?" "How do you have a successful career and a family?" "Where do you find the time?"* I do not profess to have all the answers, but I have found nuggets of wisdom that have served me well over the years. *I know that having it all does not mean having it all at once.*

I have the pleasure of being the mother to two amazing young men and the wife of a very supportive spouse who is also a pharmacist. Raising a family while also working to advance a professional career is not easy, but it can be done. I always thought I would have to give up aspects of my professional life to have a family, but that is far from the case. When I became a mom, one of my colleagues and informal mentors shared a story with me. Her mother worked throughout her childhood; however, she never missed a significant event in my friend's life. In fact, many times she was the first parent to arrive. That story gave me hope and momentum to continue knowing that I, too, could do it. *Has it been easy?* No, but it has probably been worth more to me than my boys. It has presented challenges. For example, I prepared for Utilization Review Accreditation Commission (URAC) accreditation in my car while my son took piano lessons, worked on my laptop at baseball fields throughout the Southeast, prepared for morning rounds after a 4 a.m. newborn feeding, and taken conference calls driving to a college counseling meeting. Creativity is a must when juggling a professional career and a family.

Life Balance—One cannot describe juggling career and family without mentioning the concept of work-life balance. Regardless of age, career experience or gender, many pharmacy professionals constantly struggle with finding this appropriate balance. What is funny to me is the concept itself. Think about it—balancing work and life exactly 50/50 all the time. The idea that work and life are not integrated and should share the exact same percentage of priority is a falsehood. We all have lives; work and family are simply parts of it. Life is a long journey, and your balance will tip more at times to either work or family depending on what is happening in your life at the time. Do not compartmentalize the two, but instead integrate them as much as possible. I keep one calendar where I incorporate work meetings and deadlines with family events and responsibilities. By putting all the information together, I can visualize my planning to be successful in my life. Calendar control is only one of several recommendations to find a sense of balance.

Efficiency—Organization is key to having it all. Organize your calendar, organize your desk, and organize your thoughts. Clutter takes control and robs you of the key elements of efficiency. Touch communication once—delete, trash, or respond. This applies to electronic and paper communication. My mother-in-law is in awe of how I sort the mail over the trash can. Junk mail is discarded or shredded, and bills are removed and placed in envelopes to be paid as the budget allows. Although this concept is quite natural to me, others struggle with efficient use of time.

My staff knows I am addicted to sticky notes. I have packs everywhere at work as well as at home—even in my closet! Some of my best ideas have come to me while in the shower or drying my hair! I jot down the information, place the note in a pocket on my phone case, and bring it to work to discuss. I also use this process for personal obligations. While in a meeting or answering emails, an idea or personal family issue might occur to me that will require a family discussion. Again, I make a note, place the note in my phone case, and take the note home as a reminder. Work and family thoughts will blend into your day. Accepting the thought and organizing it for the most opportune time to discuss helps with my mental work–life balance. The more disciplined you are to being efficient, the more control you will have of your time.

Communication and Planning—When planning and implementing departmental projects, you must meet with those parties involved and coordinate schedules and conflicts. The same should hold true with your personal life. My husband and I still have Sunday night meetings. We review our calendars for the following several weeks and discuss family activities and responsibilities openly. Sometimes my calendar allows me to carry more of the family load and other times my husband will. Do not keep score; simply realize that professional responsibilities vary at times during the year and contribute when and how you can.

Just Say "Yes"—A sense of balance is important, but don't overlook opportunities. Not only do we need to overcome the challenges of work and family life, but we also need to recognize the opportunities and desires in our professional lives. I have been a member of the department of pharmacy at Wake Forest Baptist Health for over 25 years. I constantly hear comments about whether you can grow and develop unless you have experienced working for other institutions. Although I agree with that concept for some individuals, it has not been the case for me. In 25 years, I have served in a multitude of roles, caring for different patient populations and leading various initiatives. *How did I do this?* I have taken advantage of opportunities placed before me no matter how different or uncomfortable they made me feel. Too many young professionals define their 5- and 10-year plans and think they can control the outcome. It is important to plan and set professional goals, but at times this narrow focus may prevent you from seeking out new experiences.

Say *"yes"* to the invitation to lead a committee, do not overanalyze the opportunity to implement a new project with a colleague in another area of pharmacy practice, and be confident to become involved in state and national pharmacy organizations. I made the decision to say "*yes*" to the previous examples, and the experiences shaped my pharmacy career for the better. I said "yes" to running for a seat on the Board of the North Carolina Association of Pharmacists, and that decision ultimately led to becoming the organization's president. Working with a colleague to implement a new service eventually led to accepting a leadership role in a new area of pharmacy practice led by that individual. Remember your professional career and goals should not be measured by the successes of those around you, but instead on the path you choose to take and the joy you find in *your* journey.

Give Back Professionally—Giving back to the pharmacy profession can also provide a sense of career balance. Instead of completing tasks and strategizing for the future, consider helping to shape the future of pharmacy by influencing new practitioners. Many years ago, I became involved with student and resident precepting and eventually this experience led me to becoming the Residency Coordinator of the PGY1 pharmacy practice residency. As a leader in the program, I contributed to the program's significant improvement and growth. Many hours were spent providing professional advice to residents, offering support, and watching them evolve into successful practitioners. I am overwhelmed with pride when I witness their ongoing successes and contributions to the profession.

This pleasure in shaping future leaders caused me to begin a PGY1 community-based pharmacy residency program; I am the Residency Program Director. Lots of work and time go into creating a new residency program. I spent many weekends planning and completing guidelines and schedules. My work life was off-balance, but now the outcomes of the program are more than I could have ever imagined. Perhaps this time could have been spent in other leadership opportunities, but I can assure you that those other experiences would not be as fulfilling.

Schedule Happiness—To avoid burnout in your career, an article I read advised scheduling "happiness." One of the recommendations was to schedule meetings throughout your day and week that bring you happiness. Whether it is having lunch with a past associate, spending 30 minutes chatting with a new department member, or participating in a webinar around a topic that interests you, these scheduled times will provide an opportunity for you to exhale and simply enjoy your day rather than dreading an upcoming two-hour planning session. I look forward to my scheduled lunch-time meetings with past direct reports and nursing associates. Schedule happiness in your day and find that balance between professional obligation and development.

Be Confident—Professional women continually need to remind them-selves to be confident when presenting or speaking with others. Women natu-rally minimize their importance by altering their body language, tone of voice, or word choice. I make a conscious effort of displaying a confident demeanor even when I may not feel overly confident. I am constantly reminded of the overuse of the word "sorry" by women, but not by men, the crossing of arms against the chest, or avoiding a seat at the conference room table. Women need to embrace their knowledge and attitude by standing tall, shaking hands, and sitting at the table. Wardrobe can also play a role in being confident. I always remind my residents to *"look good, feel good, and do good."* This doesn't mean I am dictating a dress code, but instead supporting them in making wardrobe selections that make them feel empowered. Even putting on a lab coat can make a difference.

Ask for Help—Success is not achieved alone. The saying "it takes a village" is especially important when balancing all aspects of professional and personal life. Do not be afraid to ask for help or indicate that you need it. There are no trophies for doing it all alone! Ask another mom to pick up your children, hire a sitter so you can finish that important project, or simply spend the day relaxing. Professionally, be willing to ask for clarification on an assignment or assistance running a report. We are all busy, so spending eight hours teaching yourself a software program may not be time well spent when your colleague is proficient at using the program. Again, you never know unless you ask.

"Having it all" is an unrealistic concept that we—as women—have placed on ourselves. When thinking about what that "all" includes, it also implies having everything you think you need, as well as want, all at once. The great job, the wonderful family, the loving spouse—the ideal holiday card photo. We, as successful women, have subscribed to an ideal that we will kill ourselves to achieve. *Remember that the "all" we struggle to find is out there and will come to us in phases. Get ready and enjoy the ride!*

Best,

Regina

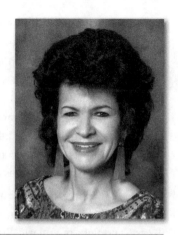

Rita Shane
PharmD, FASHP, FCSHP

Be a Brand, Not a Generic

For many people, Rita needs no introduction. A passionate and sustained leader in pharmacy, Rita exudes a strong personal brand. Her sense of individuality and zeal for stimulating change was cultivated early by her mother. Rita shares her life's guiding principles including perspectives on marriage and relationships, commitment to family, and commitment to the profession.

Rita is currently the Chief Pharmacy Officer and Professor of Medicine at Cedars-Sinai Medical Center and Assistant Dean, Clinical Pharmacy, and a Clinical Pharmacy Professor at the University of California San Francisco School of Pharmacy. Previously she was Director of Pharmacy Services at Cedars-Sinai Medical Center. She completed her pre-pharmacy coursework (1974) at the University of California Los Angeles and her PharmD (1978) at the University of Southern California.

Rita's advice is: Develop your individuality—your own brand, don't take "no" for an answer when you believe strongly in something, choose your life partner wisely to support you in your career, get involved professionally to support your growth, and make lifelong friends.

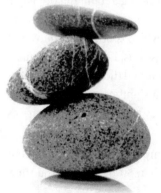

Dear Colleague,

Because many things I want to share are based on the lessons and principles I learned growing up, I will start by giving you some background. I was blessed to have a remarkable mentor, coach, and friend guide me through most of my life—my mother. She never had a chance to have an education because she was taken to Auschwitz, one of the World War II Holocaust concentration camps. However, she was a survivor, not a victim. She never talked to me about the horrors that I know she endured. Instead, she had an uncanny strength in her convictions about what was important in life which I want to share since I believe their value is timeless. She often said I was the gift that replaced what she lost; she and my father, who had a similar background, wanted to make sure that no matter what happened in this world, I would be self-sufficient. Because the war had deprived my mother of the ability to attend college, she felt very strongly about the importance of education and having a profession.

I would characterize my mother as a thoroughly modern woman who was an extremely progressive, unorthodox thinker—rare for someone born in the 1920s—and very pragmatic. Starting from my early years, probably since I was sentient, she taught me that being an individual was the most important thing for a woman. She emphasized the value of differentiating one's self rather than following what others were doing, whether it be behavior, appearance, or career choice, just for the sake of conforming. From my mother's perspective, being an individual meant having goals, having a presence, and being able to communicate effectively. She believed that it was possible to achieve anything if one was willing to put forth the effort. As I reflect on her teachings, I recognize my mother was a brand, not a generic, and she wanted me to be one also.

My mother became a seamstress when she came to the United States so she could work from home. It should be no surprise then that shopping became our favorite past time. Besides the fun we had exploring unusual possibilities of colors and clothes that looked good together, she taught me how to put myself together. She said that "it's important to have confidence in yourself which starts with your appearance, especially since you're a professional and always in the public eye." The importance of presence was especially emphasized as I was growing up: from my posture, which my mother was particularly emphatic about since I have scoliosis, to how to feel at ease entering a room full of people I didn't know. To help me develop these skills, my parents enrolled me in "charm school" when I was 15 years old. It cost them $300, which is probably equivalent to at least $3000 today. After 10 weeks of 3-hour sessions, I emerged 10 pounds lighter, learned how to gracefully enter a room, and learned the cost-effectiveness of generic versus brand name makeup. There was a significant ROI (return on investment) for the $300 program based on the money saved in future purchases of makeup alone!

On the subject of marriage and relationships, my mother had a 50 percent rule. She said that overall if you are happy more than 50 percent of the time, you have found the right partner. Basically, in any relationship, there are peaks and troughs—basic pharmacokinetic principles that have been invaluable throughout my life both personally and professionally.

Based on these guiding principles, I built my life pathway. Professionally, my "big hairy audacious goal" (see J. Collins and J.I. Porras, *Built to Last*) was and has always been to demonstrate the value of pharmacy services wherever there are patients. At the same time, my personal goal was to find a suitable partner with whom to share my life and raise a family.

Choosing a partner is probably the second most important decision in life (deciding to be a pharmacist being the first)—finding someone who will enable you to grow and develop as a total person, a professional, a parent, and a spouse or life partner. To achieve your life goals, choose your partner wisely. I still recall dating experiences where I would be enthusiastically describing some aspect of pharmacy and observe the facial expression on the person sitting across from me, which looked very much like a flatline electrocardiogram. It wouldn't have been possible to pursue my life goals without the support of a husband who has respected how important pharmacy is to my overall happiness. I have always told my residents to make sure they are clear about their career goals in discussions with prospective life partners. From my standpoint, this topic is gender agnostic. I believe that this "informed consent" approach is essential to set expectations for the future.

Being involved professionally has always been a priority in my career. When my children were young, I made the decision not to run for an office because my position as Pharmacy Director kept me quite busy and I was concerned about travel days away from home. Instead, I contributed by actively volunteering for committees at the local, state, and national levels. I believe that getting involved professionally is one of the most fulfilling aspects of our profession: it will keep you stimulated, help you build your confidence, and give you a network of advisors to support you through both your personal and professional life. My daughter says that when I go to an ASHP meeting, it's my Disneyland.

I made a commitment to my family that I would always be home for dinner, although at times, my physical presence was there but my mind was still preoc-cupied with the latest work issues. My children did a great job mentoring me to be present. They also taught me to respect how every individual is different, and the importance of listening rather than always trying to find a response. (I still need improvement in this area). My children are my best investment and my trusted advisors. I know that they have made me a better person and a better leader.

About 5 years into my role as Pharmacy Director and at a time when my children were under 10 years old, I was given the opportunity to advance to a Vice President role responsible for pharmacy, laboratory, and imaging. I realized how much I loved pharmacy and decided that rather than a "vertical" career path, I preferred to develop a "horizontal" one and set the following goals: expand professional involvement in committees at the national level, volunteer to provide presentations, and stretch myself by publishing two to three articles per year. This plan would enable me to continue developing my communication skills and staying involved professionally. The path upward in any organization is a very personal choice, and the answer lies within what makes *you* feel satisfied and happy in your career.

At work, my goal has always been to enhance the presence of my staff by finding new opportunities for pharmacists to demonstrate value. I am passionate about the need for pharmacists to continue to advance their roles, to differentiate themselves, and to create their individual "brand." I often say to my staff, "Nurses and physicians should ask for you by your name. If you are called 'pharmacy' when you are in patient care areas, it's because you haven't taken the time to let them know who you are and to demonstrate the value you bring to them and to patients." Don't let this happen to you.

As a general principle, I don't think we should accept "no" when we believe strongly in an issue related to patient care or the profession. Getting tech-check-tech programs approved by the State Board of Pharmacy took us 13 years. Throughout this time, we were repeatedly told that it would never be approved due to strong opposition by retail pharmacists who thought this would metastasize to outpatient pharmacies and reduce jobs. We continued to conduct research and share results with the Board, emphasizing that tech-check-tech programs helped pharmacists to improve medication safety in hospitalized patients by preventing prescribing and administration errors. Our outcomes, showing harm prevented by having pharmacists perform clinical functions, ultimately resulted in its approval. I have learned that being told "no" is an important lesson and an impetus to redirect one's approach, identify relevant new tactics, and whenever possible, provide compelling data. If you strongly believe in something, don't accept "no" as a response. Instead, consider what's important to stakeholders, redirect your approach, and use evidence to get to "yes."

In summary, some of my guiding principles are:

- Be a brand, not a generic.
  - o   Commit to life-long learning so you can continue to demonstrate your expertise.
  - o   Develop your presence and your communication skills.
  - o   Create a demand for your brand.
- Choose your partner wisely and invest in your family—they are your most important assets.
- Get involved professionally in the way that makes the most sense for you.
- Don't take "no" for an answer when you believe strongly in a patient care or professional issue.

Remember, we are all a work in progress and continue to learn from each other.

Wishing you all the best in a profession I hope you'll love as much as I do,

Rita

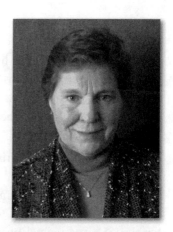

Donna Soflin
BS Pharm, FASHP

Follow Your Instincts, and Pursue Your Career with Passion and Integrity

Donna stayed committed to her rural Nebraska hospital for over 40 years and, during that time, developed a wide-ranging pharmacy practice and assumed several roles including Vice President of Quality. Donna also served on the Nebraska State Board of Pharmacy and the ASHP Board of Directors.

Donna is recently retired as Director of Pharmacy and Vice President, Quality, Lexington Regional Health Center, Lexington, Nebraska. Donna graduated from the University of Nebraska College of Pharmacy (1975) and completed an ASHP-accredited hospital pharmacy residency from the University of Nebraska Medical Center.

Donna's advice is: Be true to your values; be trustworthy, reliable, and honest; avoid gossip and judging others; be humble; lead by example; do the right thing; and simply live by the Golden Rule—a choice that is not always easy!

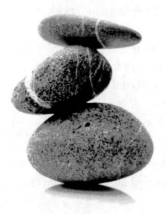

Dear Colleague,

Having recently retired after 41 years of practice in a small, rural hospital, I can happily report I had a great career there. Deciding to retire wasn't the easiest life decision, but the process followed the same pattern of decision-making I've used throughout my life and career. So I write this with the hope of lending insight that might be helpful to women in pursuit of a rewarding career in pharmacy.

141

As I summarize my career and professional activities, you will see my decision-making process has been pragmatic. My decisions were primarily based on previous experiences, gathered facts, anticipated commitment of time and effort, consideration of pros/cons, and input from colleagues and mentors. Having a crystal ball to look into the future to see the outcome of decisions before making them would be wonderful, but using the information at hand is the best one can do.

Two events occurred during my last year of college that greatly influenced my future. Half-way through the year, clerkships in various pharmacy settings broadened my view of post-graduation possibilities, but I still had no clear vision of which direction I wanted to take. In late winter I was encouraged to apply for the ASHP-accredited pharmacy residency at the University of Nebraska Medical Center. After careful consideration, I applied and was accepted into the program. At about the same time, I elected to take the first offering of a clerkship in a small, rural hospital in central Nebraska. It was my revelation! Having grown up in a rural community, I enjoyed the nonurban setting. My preceptor was a recent graduate who showed me endless opportunities that existed in the small hospital. Being the first woman to start a new, full-time hospital pharmacy service in a rural hospital in Nebraska made a huge impression on me! She was a "just get it done" person, who faced the challenge of starting a new service with persistence and patience, with little focus on barriers related to gender. The bigger barrier—one which I would also face—was starting new services among a hospital staff that had no prior exposure to a full-time pharmacist. She became one of my earliest mentors, and I credit her with helping me find my practice passion! I headed into the residency program with a clear vision of what I wanted my future practice to be.

Near the end of my residency, I was very excited to learn that a hospital administrator had contacted the college about starting pharmacy services in a soon-to-be-completed hospital in a rural Nebraska community. I quickly made contact, and a date for an interview was soon set. The hospital administrator was one of only a few female hospital administrators in the state. During the interview, we made an immediate connection. She, too, was from a rural community, was very congenial and easy going, conducted a relaxed interview, listened intently to my questions, and responded in a positive, encouraging manner. Within a week I was offered the position. I was ecstatic, as my dream appeared to be near at hand!

However, the actual decision process was a bit more complicated. I was newly married and my husband, who had just completed his degree in business administration, was also seeking employment. He had grown up in the city, but we were "on the same page" in making decisions. After due consideration, we agreed to give small-town life a try. He soon found a job, and we loaded up the U-Haul! This began my professional career as a one-person pharmacy service. I started a month before the new hospital opened to get fixtures, equipment, and supplies in place. I started the process of getting acquainted with the physicians and nurses, none of whom had any experience with a full-time pharmacist or clinical pharmacy services. I introduced them to the services and the drug distribution system I was implementing. Within a relatively short time, I felt I was a valued member of the healthcare team. Because I wanted to pay forward the opportunity to introduce students to the comprehensive pharmacy services of a small hospital, I became a preceptor for an elective rural hospital clerkship.

In small hospitals, people often wear many hats. I demonstrated a willingness to work hard, accept responsibility, and successfully complete tasks. I was proud to be tapped on several occasions to fill additional roles. There really was no decision to be made on my part, as I wasn't given the privilege of saying "no"! However, these were learning and challenging opportunities. They were somewhat stressful and time-consuming but also rewarding. These "hats" included coordinating the hospital's first three accrediting cycles with the Joint Commission, serving several years as the Regulatory Compliance Coordinator, and starting and coordinating the Patient Care and Patient Safety Committee. These added responsibilities certainly expanded my perspective of quality healthcare delivery and the role played by pharmacy services, thus influencing how services would be expanded. Becoming a leader in the administrative team evolved gradually over this time. Working primarily with women, it was important to learn the differences in how women (versus men) handle conflict, make decisions, and communicate.

Through the years I was honored to participate in professional activities outside the hospital. Soon after becoming situated in my hospital, I met other pharmacy directors from surrounding small hospitals at area meetings. These fellow pharmacy directors, female and male, from small and larger hospitals across the state, became my networking contacts. We were all willing to share our time, experience, knowledge, and wisdom with one another. As a one-person practice, this networking was invaluable. These colleagues encouraged me to join them in traveling to the Nebraska Society of Hospital Pharmacists (NSHP) meetings several times a year in Lincoln or Omaha. As usually happens in organizations, involvement starts with committee assignments and then evolves into leadership positions. I eventually served as President for NSHP, which led to involvement with ASHP. First I was appointed to an ASHP Council. I served as a Nebraska delegate to the ASHP House of Delegates, and then was honored to be elected to the ASHP Board of Directors, where I felt my contribution was my insight into the reality of pharmacy practice in a small hospital. I was also appointed by the Governor to the Nebraska Board of Pharmacy for 10 years as the hospital representative. These experiences and the colleagues I met energized and inspired me immeasurably!

My decision to participate in all these activities was made pragmatically. Any activities involving time away from work were discussed with my chief executive officer, especially since it required hiring a relief pharmacist to provide coverage. There were many personal considerations including time away from home to attend meetings and conferences, time for meeting preparation, time for travel, and financial implications. Family and personal considerations weighed heavily in every decision process. My husband was very supportive of my career and professional activities and always encouraged me to take an active part. Being DINKs (dual income, no kids) and both highly committed to our careers made balancing home/work/professional activities less complicated than for many of my colleagues.

I've often been asked why I stayed at one place for my entire career. On several occasions my husband and I considered other employment opportunities. We always weighed the perceived pros and cons for each of us. We were happy with living in a small community and were challenged and happy in our jobs. I always felt the opportunities to grow pharmacy services were endless, limited only by my own commitment and energy. Sure, there were some tough times, but they were far outweighed by the good.

Throughout the years I've learned many things that could be offered as advice. I'm not referring to things about the mechanics of pharmacy practice that continually evolve (i.e., practice models, quality initiatives, regulatory compliance, robotics, informatics), but personal integrity, experience with leadership, achieving success, and working with people.

Accountability. As the only pharmacist for 25 years, I learned that at the end of every day I was solely responsible for the day's successes, and failures, in the pharmacy service arena. It was up to me to build on the successes and learn from the mistakes.

Personality types, gender differences, generational differences, and cultural differences impact working relationships. Understanding these differences helps us understand ourselves and can significantly improve relationships with co-workers and patients.

Success. I believe the boundaries for women in the health professions have been erased, so any dream or opportunity can be successfully pursued. There are many quotes about achieving success. My favorites, which appeared on sticky notes in my office, include: "Success = hard work + perseverance + enthusiasm + humility," "Don't climb your ladder to success at the expense of another," "Destiny is not a matter of chance, but a matter of choice."

Teamwork. Effective teamwork is essential to the delivery of high-quality healthcare and customer satisfaction. Many resources are available to build teamwork skills.

Mentors and mentoring. Don't overlook the wisdom others have gained through their experiences. Find a mentor, and be open to what they offer. You may feel more comfortable with a female mentor; however, it is more important to feel comfortable and confident with your working relationship regardless of gender. Then pay it forward when you have an opportunity to mentor a student, new practitioner, or newly-hired coworker.

Be prepared. There is a lot of credibility in being prepared for meetings, conference calls, and presentations. Completion of reading or assigned tasks and reviewing agendas prior to a meeting increases productivity and shows respect for everyone's time. When coordinating a meeting, get the agenda and supporting materials distributed beforehand to the attendees; it reflects good organizational skills and time management. People appreciate that.

Leadership. I believe leadership skills are *learned*, not inherited, by following the example of leaders in our lives, participating in leadership programs, or becoming students of the multitude of resources about leadership. Willingness to serve in a leadership role is a personal decision deserving of careful consideration.

Personal integrity. Lastly, this is the trait I most value in myself and others, at work and in life. To me, integrity includes being true to one's values; being trustworthy, reliable, and honest; avoiding gossip and judging others; being humble; leading by example; doing the right thing; and simply living by the Golden Rule. It is a choice that is not always easy to make!

Follow your dreams!

Donna

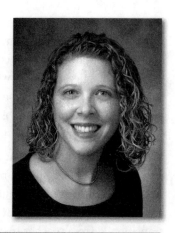

Meghan Swarthout
PharmD, MBA, BCPS

CEO of the Household—Stay-at-Home Dad

Meghan, a married young leader, outlines specific advice on how she and her husband are managing their life and family. She indicates it requires finding the right partner and believing in the inherent power you have to choose the life path that is best for you.

Meghan is currently Division Director, Ambulatory and Care Transitions, Department of Pharmacy, The Johns Hopkins Health System, Baltimore, Maryland; Residency Program Director, postgraduate year 1 and 2 (PGY1/PGY2) community health-system pharmacy administration residency; and Lecturer, Leadership and Management, University of Maryland School of Pharmacy. She received her PharmD (2009) from Ohio Northern University, Ada, Ohio and her MBA, Medical Services Management, from The Johns Hopkins Carey Business School, Johns Hopkins University. Meghan completed an ASHP-accredited PGY1/PGY2 health-system pharmacy administration residency at The Johns Hopkins Hospital.

Meghan's advice is: Communicate clearly, honestly, and often; create an accountability structure for your career and family; be clear about your priorities; and find joy and meaning in quiet, unassuming moments of life.

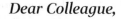

Dear Colleague,

A few months after I started dating Joey, we attended a collegiate awards program together as fellow student leaders. I received unexpected recognition that evening and was asked to stay after the program to take some photos. I got caught up in the moment and conversations; more time passed than I realized. As I finally wrapped up, I saw Joey quietly sitting in the back of the room with my purse and coat by his side. I complimented him on his purse and shoes style combo, sheepishly acknowledging my appreciation that he had patiently waited while holding my bag. He looked back with pride in his eyes and said, "I want to be the person holding your purse for the rest of your life." It was my first glimpse of what having a supportive partner really meant.

In the 10+ years since that evening, we've gotten engaged, married, and started a family. We learned how to communicate better through a two-year, long-distance relationship during residency. He moved to Baltimore after I finished my residency so I could continue to pursue a position I'm passionate about, with an organization and team that make me excited to get up every morning. He has transitioned from teacher to at-home dad, or as he aptly titled his role, CEO of the Household. Our life decision to embrace less traditional gender dynamics in our household has been met primarily with support, sometimes with surprise, and occasionally with veiled or overt criticism. Making our partnership work and striving for the elusive work–life integration requires communication, accountability, a focus on priorities, and learning to live in the moment.

Effective communication is the cornerstone of success for interpersonal interactions in all settings, perhaps none more important than at home, especially for items of great significance such as discussing possible promotions and career changes that may involve a move, as well as items of smaller significance such as who is going to wash the dishes. Speaking of dishes, we don't divide household responsibilities 50/50. I'd estimate I handle about 10 to 20% of household tasks (and that might be generous). We have to communicate how to best share the responsibilities, and I have learned that I need to be clear in communicating expectations. For example, he can't read my mind about how to do my laundry. If I want him to wash some clothes on the delicate cycle and lay sweaters flat to dry, I need to be clear!

The big topics require more longitudinal discussions. Joey and I regularly discuss my career goals and how they align with our family goals. When I have been presented with a potential career opportunity at another organization, we have transparent conversations. I have happily chosen to pursue opportunities and promotions at the same institution through this point in my career, and regular discussions and sharing of goals prevent surprises and help us make mutually agreeable decisions as a team.

Like all relationships, Joey and I have disagreements and times when our behaviors fall short of each other's expectations. This is where accountability becomes critical. For example, because it isn't possible to get home at the same time every night, it was frustrating for Joey to guess when I would be home, making it difficult to schedule dinner. He also needed breaks from toddler wrangling. The solution we found was to put a chalkboard on our kitchen wall where we write out our weekly plan, including my estimated arrival time. It creates shared accountability and doesn't keep my family guessing when I'll be home. Leaving the office at 5:00 p.m. every night isn't realistic, so I have one scheduled late night per week. It reduces the guilt of leaving at an earlier time on the other nights, and I can strategically plan to work on projects that need focused time during the one scheduled late night. We've learned it's definitely better to discuss accountability in a timely manner versus letting issues fester for too long.

I've spent more time than I should pursuing the unrealistic goal of perfection, and social media and societal norms further fuel these unattainable goals. Focusing on priorities helps reduce this noise and bring more meaning to our lives. My husband's top priority is the development and upbringing of our children, which means our house is dusty. I don't make birthday cakes from scratch, and I fall asleep without taking off my makeup. I've been encouraged by hearing from my role models that they outsource certain tasks like housecleaning. The need for outsourcing is different with one partner at home. Having an at-home spouse doesn't completely eliminate the need to consider what should be outsourced, and my husband and I both had to stop feeling guilty about hiring lawn services. We would rather spend our time together as a family on activities we enjoy versus mowing the lawn and raking leaves. Your house doesn't need to look like a spread from a magazine. Ice cream for dinner can be a fun treat when you forget to plan a meal. Some projects may be best left uncompleted (remember Stephen Covey's fourth quadrant).

When I returned from maternity leave after my first child, I quickly learned that I needed to be as productive as possible at work by focusing on priorities. That meant creating a better system to prioritize my to-do list, minimize unproductive time, and have a plan to manage my overflowing email inbox. I heard a productivity coach speak at a conference, and I asked my organization to support me working with the coach for a defined period. I outlined how the investment would benefit the organization, and my request was approved. The coach spent time observing my behaviors, providing honest feedback, and helping me implement a new task management system. It was well worth the time and money invested! If you feel like you are drowning, consider engaging an executive coach or productivity coach to help you refocus your priorities and maximize your effectiveness at work.

A key priority is making time for my relationship with Joey and ensuring care time for myself. We don't have immediate family close to us due to our decision to live out-of-state so I could pursue my career. We have learned that scheduling regular date nights is important, and we have to get creative with child care. We exchange babysitting nights with other parents and have found trusted babysitters through colleague recommendations (sometimes you can bribe a friend with a good bottle of wine). Make time for you, and let go of guilt. Work on a hobby, go to the spa, focus on a personal fitness plan, or indulge in your favorite guilty pleasure like a reality television show. This investment in *you* makes you happy, helps you take better care of others, and can enhance your productivity long term by taking time to decompress.

While writing a draft of this letter, my toddler asked me to play indoor bowling with water bottles and a rubber ball (try it. . . it's pretty fun). Did it put me off my timeline for task completion? *Yes.* Was it worth staying up later after he went to bed to enjoy the moment of play with him? *Absolutely.* Integration always requires decisions with trade-offs. Perfection is an illusion. *Enjoy the ordinary moments that make life special.* Create "no technology" time, such as at the dinner table and during set hours on the weekends. Shut off your email when you are out of the office.

I noted earlier that our more nontraditional gender roles are sometimes met with veiled or overt criticism. At first, we internalized these comments and didn't discuss them with each other or others. Holding in this frustration wasn't healthy. We've learned to assert ourselves more positively through the years. When someone asks Joey if he's babysitting, he proudly tells them that he's parenting. When someone asks when he's going back to work, he reminds them he works every day caring for our family. When someone asks me if I feel guilty making my husband do the housework, I tell them how proud I am to show my children that women can be senior leaders. It's not always easy, and you need a support system of people who understand and listen without judgment. Joey belongs to a national network of at-home dads. It's opened his eyes to a broader level of inclusivity, such as two-dad households, and reminds him he isn't alone. My next goal is that we stop referring to all daytime activities with the title of "Mommy and Me" and "Mom Playdates." It makes working mothers feel guilty that they can't participate and at-home fathers feel like they aren't included. Gender-neutral terms work well for all parents.

Choosing to have an at-home partner was the right decision for my family. There are many models that work, and the best model for you may be very different. You may choose to stay home, pause your career, and return to the workplace at the time that is right for you. You may have a two-career household. You may choose to pursue job-sharing and part-time work to care for children or aging parents. You may choose not to have children and care for others in your family, your friends, or the community in important ways. We need to embrace all pathways and be role models for future generations by celebrating diverse life decisions.

Ultimately, the best piece of advice I can give you, albeit a little cheesy, is to live your life as a love letter—to your patients, your team, your community, your family, and yourself. Be patient and kind to yourself and others. Communicate clearly, honestly, and often; create an accountability structure for your career and family; be clear about your priorities; and find joy and meaning in quiet, unassuming moments of life. Let's all free ourselves of our self-inflicted guilt and express more gratitude for what is working well. Be selective in finding the right partner, and know the inherent power you have in choosing the life path that is best for you.

Let's continue to break down stereotypes and inappropriate and outdated social norms. I look forward to creating a future together where there is equal gender representation in the chief executive suites and in the home.

Kind regards,

Meghan

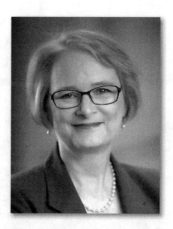

Linda Tyler
PharmD, FASHP

Figuring Things Out Along the Way

Linda's career is an example of a clinical pharmacist somewhat reluctantly moving into formal leadership while successfully managing a family. She traces the four practice specialties she has had and provides practical advice on juggling her career and life along the journey.

Linda is currently Chief Pharmacy Officer, University of Utah Health Care, Salt Lake City, Utah and Associate Dean, Pharmacy Practice, College of Pharmacy, and Professor of Pharmacotherapy (Clinical), Department of Pharmacotherapy, University of Utah. Previously she was Administrative Director and Associate Professor, Department of Pharmacy Practice, College of Pharmacy. She received her BS in Pharmacy and her PharmD (1981) from the University of Utah, College of Pharmacy. Linda completed a residency in hospital pharmacy practice at the University of Nebraska Medical Center, Omaha, Nebraska.

Linda's advice is: **YABTYK. You are better than you know. When you question and doubt yourself, it is not whether you make the *right* decision, but that you**

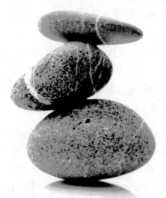

make <u>a</u> decision, the best at the time, and have the courage to make a change if it doesn't work or if other opportunities present themselves. You have more strength, courage, and abilities than you know.

Dear Colleague,

Several years ago one of my residents asked me, *"How did you do it all? How did you make career and family work?"* I responded, "You just do; you figure it out along the way." Then I realized, she was really asking! She was going to have to do this in her career.

I have practiced in four different specialties in my career: critical care, poison control, drug information, and administration. One was my choice, one was to follow my husband in his career, and one was to make a move that would be good for both of us. The last was an unexpected opportunity within my current organization. I have taken some crazy risks. If it didn't work, I regrouped and tried something else. It all worked out in better ways than I could have imagined. You have to be willing to make a change. This takes courage.

I did a residency because I was scared to find a job that, at the time, I thought would be for the rest of my life. One day, while waiting for my advisor, I noticed a flyer on the bulletin board, "Do a residency, one year." I thought to myself, *I could do anything for one year.* Because my experience as an intern was in chain stores, I figured acceptance was a long shot. In my residency, I discovered that I wanted to pursue a career in a health system so I would need my doctor of pharmacy degree. I applied to many programs, had one interview, and got accepted.

After finishing graduate school, I wanted to be a high-powered clinician, working in a fast-paced clinical environment for a college of pharmacy. I ended up with my dream job. I was well prepared for the teaching and clinical aspects, but not as well trained for scholarly activities. After a few years, I realized something needed to change. I either needed to get new skills or to change positions. But something changed for me. My husband had an opportunity in a different city. I took a position in a poison control center, throwing my energies into developing in this new position. After a year, our daughter was born. Children give you perspective on what is *really* important. I knew for me, I would not be able to return to work full time.

After a couple of years, my husband's position was not working out. We teamed up to figure out our next move. One requirement was that it needed to be closer to family, and we both found jobs in Salt Lake City. I landed in a drug information position. After a couple of years in that position, my son was born. He arrived a month early, and I had severe complications. I had to be out three months and return to work slowly over the next four months. This is not what I had planned! I had to focus on getting better and taking care of my children. I had to figure out new ways of doing things by adjusting my personal expectations and career trajectory.

The next few years were all about going to work, coming home, and spending time with my children and husband. We did no extra things. Even grocery shopping was a challenge. We kept things really simple. We make friends easily, which helps in building a stronger support network. We didn't go anywhere after work where we couldn't take our children. Every day was a puzzle; you figure out the plan for the day and hope nothing is derailed. It was like a luge run—going down the mountain, head first, keeping my fingers crossed that no one flinched. A flinch meant a spectacular crash and burn, but we would adjust and figure it out. Even when things seemed dire, there was always someone able to help, and so it was important to be there for someone else.

For 22 years, I served as Director of Drug Information Services. I loved the mix of solving clinical and organizational problems. Although my title was "Director," we had relatively few staff. However, our work spanned the entire organization. As I developed in my specialty, I became more involved with ASHP. I served on the Clinical Section when it first formed. When my daughter was 10 and my son was 7, I was invited to serve on a Council. However, Council week was the same week as both of my children's birthdays. Since the meeting was always scheduled for that week, it would always be a conflict. I discussed it with my family, explained the opportunity, and that it involved missing their birthdays. When I suggested that we could celebrate on the weekend, my daughter started to sniffle and said that I really couldn't miss their birthdays. My son, always the negotiator, touched her arm and said, "You know if we let mom go, she will probably do anything for us." My daughter thought about it, brightened, and said, "Okay, you can go." As it turned out, I only missed two of their birthdays, but my son's recollection as an adult is that I missed more often than not. This is a great example of how we always talked about things as a family and worked them out. We preserved dinner as a time for coming together.

I had actually put my name in for Board of Directors but was not slated. Although disappointed, I knew there would be other opportunities. About a year later, I was thankful it had not worked out. My kids were in junior high, and I needed to spend more time at home.

The realization was dawning that I needed to take care of myself. I had that moment where my doctor told me I needed an exercise plan. I groaned. *How was I going to do this?* That evening, my children's soccer league called and asked, "Do you want to be a soccer referee?" I said "yes," thinking it would be better than jogging alone. I ended up liking it. Being the referee meant I had to leave work on time. It made me think about something else besides work. When I was on the soccer field, I guarantee you I was not thinking about work. Although more juggling was involved, it also meant I had to make smarter decisions about both home and work, and what was really important. The result was that I slept better!

Many years later, I was talking with a friend at a national meeting. I said that I got behind when I was on maternity leave, when my son was born, and I had not caught up. Another person asked, "How old is your baby?" I replied, "22." She said that 22 months was such a fun age. I elaborated, "22 years." I gave up the notion of being caught up long before. I had to set priorities and make choices. You have to forgive yourself for not getting everything done. If you are really engaged in your job and invested in your career, you will see all kinds of possibilities. However, you will never be able to do them all, so it is important to be realistic—learn how to say "no" effectively or negotiate the deadline.

In 2008, I became the Interim Director of Pharmacy. I was a clinician and was really happy with my current role. I was a good crisis manager and would help get everyone through this interval. After six months, the Chief Operating Officer (COO) asked me to apply for the position. I said, "You know I don't want the position; this is not a position I am prepared for." He asked that I think about it. As interim, I had the opportunity to solve different problems that allowed me to connect at another level in the organization. If the COO had faith in me, maybe I should give it a try. *But what could he possibly see in me?*

I had underestimated several things. Few people had the experience I did of interfacing between the health system and the college of pharmacy. What I hadn't really realized through my career voyage was that I developed leadership skills. No one labeled the things I did as leadership. My skills at influencing— long-rooted in high school debate—were applicable to the position. Most things I did in my work and with ASHP involved leadership skills. My experiences had given me a rich foundation for the position. Someone told me early in my career that if clinicians weren't willing to take formal leadership roles, then how would clinical pharmacy practice advance? I just didn't think that someone would be *me.* So, I began to think that perhaps I should take the chance.

I was pretty overwhelmed in my new role. My new favorite word was, "Yet." So often I would feel like I couldn't do something, but then I would say I couldn't do it yet. *Yet* gave me permission that I didn't have to do everything at once, and I didn't have to know everything. I could ask for help. I would figure it out.

I am currently in the right position doing the right things. My path was not smooth or even. I am still on a steep learning curve. I couldn't have predicted where I would end up. *I offer you the following additional advice:*

- **Take care of yourself.** You will not be there to take care of those around you if you don't take care of yourself.

- *Have the courage to make a change, both in your career and your home life.* It is easy to just keep going along. But sometimes, it just creeps up on you—you are really not happy with what you are doing or what you are doing is not working. Be it your job, career, home life, or other, you just need to make the change. Life is too short not to be happy. You have options.

- *Be flexible.* You, your loved ones, and your co-workers will crash sometimes when the first plan doesn't work. You will have alternatives, and you are often figuring it out as you go along. This is not always your first instinct. Adjusting to new things, new realities, and new ideas is really important. It can open doors. Your ability to be flexible and work as a team member will define your success.

- *Imagine the possibilities.* Have a bias for yes. My husband says I am persistently, relentlessly, optimistic. Optimism is an important leadership trait. Early in my career I was persistent in doing things well, and doing them better. This overly critical view could be perceived as pessimism. I realized that negativity would sap my energy, and I didn't have any extra energy to spare. Positivity becomes really energizing.

YABTYK. *You are better than you know.* My husband started saying this to our daughter when she was in junior high. What happens in the teenage years that cause girls, in particular, to doubt themselves and their ability to take risks? Yet, when I think back, it has happened so many times in my life. We question and doubt ourselves. It is not whether we make the *right* decision, but that we make *a* decision, the best at the time, and have the courage to make a change if it doesn't work or other opportunities present themselves. We have more strength, courage, and abilities than we know.

We make a difference and serve as role models in other people's lives in ways we don't always recognize. No one sees the extreme juggling that we do to balance our rich, multidimensional lives. When the doubts creep in, remember that YABTYK. You have the strength and courage to figure it out.

Yours,

Linda

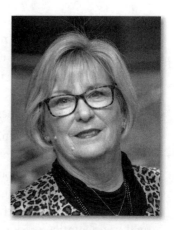

Julie Webb
BS Pharm

Have a Job That You Love

Julie shares her journey including how she and her husband have agreed that when trying to balance life and work—so everyone can enjoy equal success—the secret is for both of them to give 100%. They have made an agreement that they will contribute equally by keeping things moving without keeping score. Their focus is always on what needs to be done today to be successful tomorrow and beyond.

Julie is currently Senior Vice President, Office of Professional Development, and was previously Vice President, Office of Resources Development at ASHP in Bethesda, Maryland. She received her BS Pharm (1980) from University of North Carolina, Chapel Hill, North Carolina. Julie completed a hospital pharmacy residency at the Medical University of South Carolina, Charleston, South Carolina.

Julie's advice is: **Find your passion and you will never feel like your job is "work"; instead, you will think of your career as an enjoyable adventure. Don't be afraid to try career options that are outside your comfort zone. Always examining your life and the directions you are headed positions you to find your passion.**

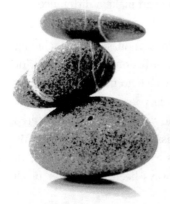

Dear Colleague,

I have a job that I love, so I really do not think of anything I do as "work." Some of the key things that have allowed me to be in this position include good luck, a commitment to discovering what contributions I could make to the profession, an equal opportunity marriage, artful mentors, and giving my all on a daily basis. By accident I became a pharmacist; by good fortune I became a member of the ASHP senior leadership staff. Being in the right place at the right time was a gift, but learning how to always make a difference was an imperative I learned from the leaders who came before me. I am writing to share my story with the hope that it will inspire another young woman to find her path to a leadership position and enjoy her career as much as I have mine.

As for the luck, I have enjoyed my share of it, but it began when I entered the University of North Carolina in Chapel Hill as a freshman. I was a strong science student in high school and decided to declare pharmacy as my major. The idea came from my roommate who was doing the same. Well, that and the fact that I did not want to give up one of my first days as a college student to attend an orientation session. I thought attending a double-header at the baseball stadium was a better choice in Chapel Hill on a beautiful fall day. I asked my roommate to bring back the registration information for pre-pharmacy so I could instead orient myself on how to attend a college sports event. That was fortuitous because I was not sure what a pharmacist actually did on a daily basis, but I was certainly comfortable with all the subject areas required.

Seeking out an advisor from the school of pharmacy was how I began the journey. I became a pharmacist, and my roommate ended up becoming an accountant. I really enjoyed the years I spent in pharmacy school and realized that I had found something I could be passionate about as a career. In my final year, one of my professors suggested that I consider doing an ASHP-accredited residency program, which seemed like an excellent way to gain some valuable experience in a short period of time. I secured a position as a hospital pharmacy resident at the Medical University of South Carolina in Charleston, South Carolina. Since you are reading this, I assume you have already chosen pharmacy as your profession. You have made a terrific choice, but choosing a profession that will inspire you to be your best is just the first step to becoming a leader. Within that profession, you will want to explore where you can make a difference and contribute in ways that will allow your leadership skills to shine.

After completing the residency, I practiced in several settings including hospital pharmacy, veterinary medicine, and home infusion. I also worked for a pharmaceutical company briefly. One piece of advice is to not be afraid to try nontraditional practice settings even if it is outside your comfort zone. Only by exploring various options can you begin to find your passion. I discovered mine could be realized when I made the leap to association management. My journey to becoming a leader began by serving as a staff member of my own professional organizational home, ASHP. I had always been an admirer of all things ASHP beginning in my student days, which certainly grew stronger when I was completing an ASHP-accredited residency. Years later I was practicing in home infusion when ASHP appointed an advisory group to determine the resources necessary to support the group's professional development needs. The then-ASHP President, now ASHP Chief Executive Officer, and my current boss, Paul Abramowitz, appointed me to the ASHP home care advisory group. I didn't know him personally, but someone who knew us both recommended me for the appointment after I submitted my name for consideration. I remind Dr. Abramowitz frequently that it was his own doing nearly 25 years ago that led to him having to deal with me on a continuous basis today. That group eventually became the Interim Executive Committee of the first ASHP section when the Section of Home Care Practitioners was launched. When the ASHP staff person who managed that Section left ASHP, I joined the staff to fill the vacancy.

I travel often to ASHP national meetings, meetings of ASHP affiliates, and other professional gatherings where I meet pharmacists who tell me they are ASHP members. My response is that I work for them and, in saying that, I am acknowledging where I have been able to make a meaningful contribution to the profession. Serving our profession as a member of the ASHP staff is something I am humbled to have been doing for most of my work life. Leading the educational enterprise at ASHP and shepherding the successes of the staff in our office is one of the most enjoyable things to me. I still get excited to go to work every day and find that I am inspired by our members, our staff, and other stakeholders in moving our profession forward. Being a leader at ASHP is easy because I truly found my passion. Finding your passion can set you free in your leadership journey.

I mentioned earlier that my marriage is a true equal opportunity adventure. Having a great life mate is critical if you want to aspire to be a leader in the profession. What I didn't mention earlier is that my husband is also a pharmacist. But the similarity in our professional life doesn't end there. His career for the last 30 years has been dedicated to serving as an association executive for other pharmacy groups. Observing his early tenure in association management was an inspiration for me. His expertise is different than mine. He focuses his efforts on policy, regulations, and legislation in healthcare where I focus on education and product development. Our specific positions are not competitive per se, but the associations we work for certainly are competitive in a business sense. This means some areas of our work lives require a firewall. One might even say that I sleep with the frenemy. I am often asked how we have maintained that firewall and had a successful marriage for 37 years. Managing such a conflict of interest (including the perceptions of some who might not appreciate that we are doing so) requires mutual respect for our chosen professional roles and recognizing that, although we may not be able to discuss certain business plans or strategic directions, we both work to move the practice of pharmacy to higher levels.

I have also been asked by students, residents, and others about how I managed to travel for work and be available for national meetings, board meetings, and other non-negotiable time commitments and *still* have a strong family commitment and relationship—in essence to "have it all." The question of balancing work and family life often becomes the focus in conversations with friends and colleagues. When a discussion of how couples split the work load to manage on a daily basis includes reports of 50/50, 60/40, or other splits, I am always the outlier when I report my family split. Our view, an absolute necessity for everyone involved to enjoy equal success, is to give 100%/100%. We have made an agreement that we will contribute equally by keeping things moving without keeping score. Instead we have always focused on what needs to be done today to be successful tomorrow and beyond. In the professional realm, we each have our areas of expertise where sometimes we stand alone and other times I am recognized as his wife or he as my husband. Our son is also a pharmacist who has begun his own professional journey in a management role at a major teaching institution. That means that we are sometimes acknowledged not because of our own roles, but as his parents. No matter the situation, we have all become comfortable and secure in how we are recognized at the time. We are the best cheerleaders for one another, and that inspires us all.

It is important to recognize the value of seeking mentors while also making a commitment to being one yourself. Student pharmacists and new graduates often think of the profession as being very large. In actuality, pharmacy is one of the smaller health professions; the more involved you become in the profession, the smaller it becomes. Be sure to value all relationships and experiences. Be careful to not burn any bridges along the way because today's challenge might just become tomorrow's opportunity.

Early in my career at ASHP, I was fortunate to have as my supervisor the Chief Operating Officer, Mary Jo Reilly. Mary Jo was an artful mentor. She knew when to offer advice and counsel and when to let me learn valuable lessons on my own. She referred to me as a great confessor because I was very comfortable bounding into her office to report on something I had done where things had not gone as expected. We would talk about what I might have done differently to achieve a different outcome. I felt safe and was not defensive in these conversations because of the trust in our relationship. As a result I began to be more and more comfortable in honest self-reflection. Looking back, I now recognize that the guidance from her allowed me to become more accountable to myself and others. The result led to my becoming a better team player by focusing on the organization's goals rather than my own goals—thus beginning my journey as a leader. Although Mary Jo retired many years ago, I still reach out to her often for advice and counsel especially when I find myself in a difficult situation. She has an innate ability to help me find solid ground and make emotionally intelligent decisions. In turn, I have worked to become a mentor in my own right, but I recognize that I may never be able to attain the same skills. However, I continue to develop trusting relationships with those I mentor and provide some valuable guidance along the way.

Always examining your life and the directions you are headed positions you to find your passion. Being a leader follows naturally when you are making choices which allow that passion to grow. Keep looking until you find yours, and you will wake up one morning and realize someone is looking up to you and what you have to offer as valuable even if you accidentally arrived at your current destination!

Find your passion,

Julie

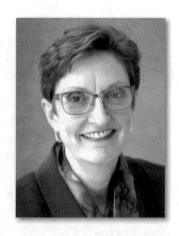

Valorie Wilkins
BS Pharm, MS, MBA, MHIHIM

Lead from Where You Are

Val shares her experiences and lessons from moving around the country for her career, practicing in different settings, and completing several graduate degrees. She is reinventing herself and thriving after surviving a layoff and cancer.

Val is currently Clinical Pharmacist, Cascade Valley Hospital, Arlington, Washington, and Faculty, Pharmacy Leadership Academy, Course 5 Leading Transformational Change. Previously she was Director of Pharmacy, Swedish Edmonds (formerly Stevens Hospital), Edmonds, Washington. Val received her BS in Pharmacy from the University of Washington, Seattle, Washington. She completed an ASHP-accredited hospital pharmacy residency, North Carolina Memorial Hospital; an MS from the University of North Carolina, Chapel Hill, North Carolina; an MBA from the Executive Development Program, William E. Simon Graduate School of Business Administration, University of Rochester, Rochester, New, York; and her MHIHIM from the School of Public Health, University of Washington, Seattle.

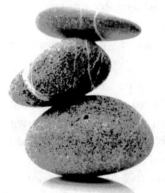

Val's advice is: What I know now is that we cannot succeed as clinicians or leaders if we're in positions that do not harmonize with our basic beliefs about who we are and what we do.

Dear Colleague,

Lead from where you are—even if where you are isn't where you thought you'd be. My path originally seemed straightforward. I had learned early that pharmacy was for me. The connection and interplay between biology and chemistry fascinated me, and when I discovered pharmacy, that was it! I went straight from high school into pre-pharmacy at the University of Washington in Seattle.

Hospital pharmacy was always my goal; after graduation with my BS in Pharmacy I was matched via ASHP to the combined Residency/Master's program at the University of North Carolina at Chapel Hill. I moved thousands of miles away from home to a place where I knew no one and even the food was different. I still remember my first breakfast at the hospital—there were things on the steam table (grits and hominy) that I'd only read about in books; I was very young. North Carolina taught me that there were good people everywhere who were willing to teach if you were willing to learn.

Then it was on to Rochester, New York, where I discovered matrix management and snow. As the Pharmacy Medicine Service Chief, I was in charge of pharmacy services to a defined section of the hospital and the matrix management structure meant that I represented the department in multidisciplinary settings. Observing how physician leaders handled the medicine service line made me curious about pharmacy as a business, and I asked the department to sponsor me in an Executive MBA program. Rochester also taught me lateral leadership and if I never missed a plane, I was getting to the airport too early (advice from a former head of the Securities and Exchange Commission).

Family drew me back to Seattle, and I took a job managing the first freestanding infusion suite for a national firm. It was a wonderful opportunity to finish the build-out and opening of our physical space as well as creation of a new clinical and business model. We provided a quality service, and I had no difficulty with the business aspects—except for marketing. The company sent me to corporate sales school, and while I grasped the concepts, they didn't feel right. Having come from a multidisciplinary team environment, I wasn't comfortable "selling" one venue as the single best spot for patients to receive care, and eventually began to question the direction of the business model. Revenue seemed more important than patient outcomes, and I struggled with the mismatch between my personal values and my professional role.

When I was offered an opportunity to move back to the company's base business of home infusion, I jumped at the chance. It took me a fair amount of time to feel ready to step into another management position because I felt that I'd failed as a team leader. In retrospect, and more realistically, it was a bad match. What I know now is that we cannot succeed as clinicians or leaders if we're in positions that do not harmonize with our basic beliefs about who we are and what we do. Take the time early in your career to reflect on your personal values and their professional implications as well as your hopes and dreams. You will rely on those reflections if you find yourself in a similar situation.

While I was still in my "I'm not ready to be a leader again" phase, I experimented with a number of pharmacy settings working as an agency pharmacist. It can be easy to be dismissive of professionals who prefer term contract or agency work, but I can tell you that it takes a great deal of skill. I learned to value a pharmacist's contributions to care in practice settings that I'd never worked in previously, as well as learning other important lessons. Agency pharmacists walk into a work environment "cold." Because your skills will almost always be underestimated, you need to check your ego at the door. You must quickly work to establish firm relationships so you can function as part of a new group; something I now know as *teaming*. In this environment, extreme teaming demands tightly honed skills.

One of the hospitals bought my contract from the agency, and I went back to hospital pharmacy. Less than a year after I'd become a fulltime employee, I was the Interim Director of Pharmacy—two weeks before our scheduled Joint Commission visit. No pressure!

I stayed with the organization for 16 years, working as a Staff Pharmacist, Clinical Coordinator, and Director, with a couple of stints as Acting Director. We had a wonderful team that accomplished a great deal; I was proud to be the Director of Pharmacy. On the surface I seemed to be at the pinnacle of my personal goals but as the organization changed so did my job satisfaction. Then I was unexpectedly called to my boss's office and told that my position was being eliminated—they were combining the Ambulatory and Inpatient Director positions. Strangely enough, my first emotion at the time was relief as I thought *I don't have to do this anymore*. Then I went into shock; it felt as though my family had been amputated.

Layoffs are hard—you just vanish, and people may not be told why you're gone. You become something of a professional pariah; former staff and colleagues don't know how to talk to you even if they have your contact information, all of which leaves you angry, lonely, and feeling like you're in a sort of quarantined purgatory.

I won't kid you, it was tough, but later I realized that it was probably the best thing that had happened to me in years. The position and the organization had changed over time, and I'd been so busy doing my job that I'd missed the slow divergence between my personal values and my professional role. I'd slowly become increasingly unhappy with my position. If I hadn't been laid off, I don't think I would have ever left the people who I thought depended on me. I'd probably still be there, overworking myself right into continued poor health.

I'd maintained my clinical skills by working as an on-call pharmacist for a friend who was a director at a small community hospital. So, I spent the next few months working part time, pulling some shifts there, getting my head together, and thinking things over. A friend advised me to savor my time off; that I would regret going back to work too soon. He was right—I hadn't had more than 2½ weeks off in a row since I'd graduated from the University of Washington and was studying for Boards.

Taking time for myself was new and uncomfortable at first, but it allowed me to think about the things that I liked and things that frustrated me in my previous positions. I rediscovered my love for pharmacy and realized that my values and skills were part of *me* and not the positions I held. And the house got really clean.

Trolling the Internet one day I found an interesting Master's program in Health Informatics and Health Information Management at the University of Washington. I was immediately intrigued because I've always been a self-described data-junkie and incredibly frustrated by the phrase "Epic doesn't have a report for that." I'd long felt that it was time the computers worked for us—instead of us for them.

I applied to the program, took a full-time position at the hospital where I was working, and went back to being a student. I'm not sure if I'd forgotten how hard it was to go to school full-time and work full-time, or if I'd just deluded myself that it wouldn't be that hard, but it took some adjusting. I was the oldest student in my cohort, and I think my classmates despaired over my lack of technical skills; I was a techno-dinosaur. I like to joke that it was Val version 2.0 that graduated. My cohort was small, and we became close; my study group became another family. That turned out to be incredibly important, because in October, two months into our second year, I was diagnosed with endometrial cancer.

My life is now neatly divided in two—before cancer and after cancer. I was lucky; I staged at 1B. My surgery and optional radiation were completed by the start of January. I went back to school (we did one on-site weekend a month) 9 days post-op and to work at 14 days. Not my best decision ever, even with a robotic surgery. The pain wasn't bad, but the exhaustion was crippling. My study group and family helped to paste me back together, and we went forward. But it was very difficult. I should have known better and taken more time off.

I finished my degree, completing the program with my cohort, but things didn't go quite as I'd expected after graduation. I had envisioned working on the bridge between clinicians/patients and technology, but cancer has changed my life in more than one way during the last year.

I have an autoimmune arthritis and had begun exploring ways to modify my diet and health behaviors even before I was laid off. While I was deciding what to do next, I continued that process. I'd had some success but fell back into bad habits with full-time school and work. Cancer changed that for me completely. Suddenly facing your own mortality is a wonderful motivator. I did more research and made significant changes. As a result, my physical appearance changed dramatically, and people started to ask me how I'd done it. At that point, I realized that while I'd like to help the people asking me those questions, I didn't know how. I'm currently enrolled in a program to become a Functional Medicine Certified Health Coach.

My year of cancer was hard, but what they don't tell you is that the next year, when you're supposed to have your life back together, it is even harder. What's important has changed, and I'm still not sure what shape the pieces will eventually make, but I've realized that's part of the journey. My heart will always belong to pharmacy, but I may use those skills in a different way. My recent experiences as a patient gave me new understanding of what it's like to want more of a voice in my care than I was allowed. Teaching continues to be important to me, but I do it differently now that I truly understand why we must meet students where they are and not where we might want them to be. *Regardless of where my path takes me next, the following core set of values is coming with me:*

- *Take care of yourself* because no one else will do it for you. Leave enough "you" to take home.

- *Instead of work–life balance, consider strengthening your core* so that you can flex in the needed direction, be it work, family, or community.

- *Know your strengths and use them.* Don't try to gain ALL the skills you don't have. We are not superwomen; leverage the skills you have into new tools.

- *Ask for help* when you need it, and give it when you can.

- *Build family that supports and enriches who you are.* We all have many families—those we were born with, and the ones that we choose.

- *Establish relationships based on who people are*, not what they can do for you. Don't be the manager who never speaks to anyone not leading a department; everyone is important to your organization's mission.

- *Be yourself.* If the fit is poor, don't kill yourself to stay there. Get out before you're pushed.

- *Apologize, get over it, and do better.* Know that we all make mistakes at some point and hurt people unintentionally.

- *Never stop learning.* You never know what direction it will take you.

- *Expect failure.* It's not who you are, it's how you find the next step.

And finally, know that it's not a title or a position that makes you a leader, it's how you live and work. You demonstrate leadership through your actions even during times when you may not feel capable of being in charge of more than the lunch menu.

Remember the core values and skills you've built along the way, and always be excited about the possibility of re-inventing yourself to lead from where you are now.

Always stay true to yourself,

Val

Beth Steinbeck Williams
PharmD

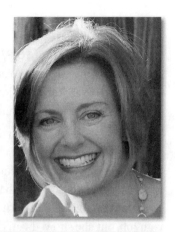

Follow Your Own Path—Titles Don't Always Matter

Beth steps back from her two-decade career and shares her unique life–career journey with its twists and turns so that others may benefit from her experiences and lessons. She is very candid, which makes this letter so powerful, and demonstrates there is not just one way for a pharmacy career and life to play out.

Beth is currently Assistant Director of Pharmacy–Population Health at Wake Forest Baptist Health, Winston-Salem, North Carolina. Previously she served as Interim Director and Director of Pharmacy. Beth received her PharmD (1996) from the University of North Carolina at Chapel Hill and completed an ASHP-accredited pharmacy practice residency at Wake Forest University Baptist Medical Center, Winston-Salem, North Carolina.

Beth's advice is: Life–career balance—a true 50/50 alignment—is not achievable. Instead, you will need to aim for harmony between your personal and professional roles.

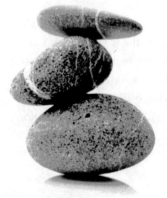

Dear Colleague,

When asked to write this letter, I decided to offer my advice via a letter to my younger self. In this way, I hope to impart guidance and wisdom that you can take on your own personal journey.

Shall we?

Dear 26-Year-Old Me,

I'm writing to you from 2018, 22 years in the future. I know it's weird, but I've got a lot of things to share. You are going to have an amazing career and family, so get ready! Well into your journey, you will receive a beautiful gift . . . you will discover who you really are and what's truly important to you.

Here you are, newly married and launching your career in your dream job, providing ambulatory care services in a small North Carolina community. It's perfect for you—building relationships and helping people. Wasn't it wonderful when Miss Lowry gave you that handmade quilt and called you her "earth-angel" to thank you for helping with her medicines? You thought you were just doing your job, but she showed you that you are making a difference! It's a gift you will cherish forever.

In a couple of years, you will move for your husband's job, and there will be an opportunity with the North Carolina Association of Pharmacists (NCAP). You will work alongside North Carolina pharmacists and replicate a community-based pharmaceutical care model in several areas of the state. It's going to be a tremendous opportunity to improve patient care, advance the profession, and build a professional network like you could never imagine. Unfortunately, you will spend only two years in this role, and you will not have an opportunity to see your work come to fruition. You see, during your time at NCAP, you will become a mom. *I know, right?!* This is only year 3 of 5, and starting a family was not in your 5-year plan. But God has a different plan in store for you.

When your son is nearly 1 year old, your husband's job will take him away from home more and more. You're going to realize that, as much as you love what you're doing at NCAP, it's just not realistic to continue commuting an hour and a half to work. You will need to make a change for your family. It won't be easy, but good news ... you will have no preconceived ideas about your next pharmacy venture, and the world is your oyster!

Note to Self: Being a mom and a professional is actually going to be harder than you anticipate and much harder than other women make it look. Let's face it; you are a workaholic by nature. Although you will not realize it, you are at a point in your life where your work defines you. It's also what you enjoy. You are deeply satisfied when you are working and serving others, and for whatever reason, you have a bend toward serving professionally. Just own it, and don't apologize for it. It's all part of the journey!

When you leave NCAP, you will reach out to Ron Small, the Director at the hospital where you did your pharmacy practice residency. I'm still not sure what you were thinking, but for some reason, you think you might be a good fit for one or two positions he is recruiting for at Wake Forest Baptist (WFB). Ron will present you with another opportunity, and you will apply for an Assistant Director position leading pharmacy satellite operations. Of course, you will technically not be qualified for this role, but that is the beauty—or blindness—of naivety. To this point in your career, you have been responsible for a program and yourself. Period. In this new role, you will be responsible for services that you haven't thought about since your residency, not to mention managing 60 people. But Ron will see something in you that you do not yet see in yourself (and he will mentor you for many years). Here is the awesome thing about this whole Assistant Director situation: *You Actually Think You Can Do It*. And you will be right. You will join the WFB pharmacy leadership team, and you will be successful because you will be surrounded by awesome people and driven to make a difference.

As much as you enjoy the role and responsibility, you will soon realize you need help if you want to implement the types of programs and services that you envision. So you will create some manager roles and begin developing the team. You will not realize you have these skills, but you *do*. You will get used to pushing yourself outside of your comfort zone. Some experiences will be exciting, and some will continue to be uncomfortable. But you will grow in the uncomfortable places.

Three years after your arrival at Wake, your second child will be born. This will be a complete game-changer. You will recall a conversation with a mentor who is a working-mom who said "when it comes to children, 1 + 1 equals 3." And she is SO RIGHT because you will feel like you need at least six hands and another brain! But you will figure it out. As much as you will be head-over-heels in love with your sweet daughter, you will also look forward to returning to work because that is where you feel most alive. In an unexpected turn of events, you will find yourself in the role of Director of Pharmacy. *Yep, I know*. You will think I'm totally making this up, because it's so inconceivable. At first, you will not even consider applying, but after a careful candidate search, it seems that you may be a good fit so you will go for it!

Note to Self: Work–life balance will be critical to both your success and survival. After several years of trying to achieve balance, a wise man will offer insight that will be life-changing. He will tell you that if you work full time, you will spend two-thirds of your waking hours at work, which means you only have one-third of your waking hours for family and self. In other words, balance—a true 50/50 alignment—is not achievable. Instead, you will need to aim for *harmony* between your personal and professional roles. As silly as it sounds, this one word will give you permission to stop aiming for something that's not achievable and will completely change the way you think about work–life balance. All because of a single word!

I don't have time to teach you everything you need to know about taking responsibility for the whole department. You will need a lot of patience, help, humility, and coffee. You will not realize it, because you don't see differences like other people do, but the fact that you are a female, in your mid-30s, and leading the pharmacy department at a large academic medical center will be of great interest to many people. They will be watching, probably trying to see if you can handle all the responsibility. It certainly won't be easy, and you'll make plenty of mistakes. But it will be some of the most rewarding years of your professional career. At first, you will try to live up to everyone's expectations because you are still in the habit of people-pleasing. But as you settle in to the role and realize the responsibility that's been given to you, you will simply strive to do what's right. The greatest lessons you will learn are the importance of seeking first to understand (*thank you, Stephen Covey*) and surrounding yourself with people you trust (i.e., people who will tell you what you don't always want to hear).

Note to Self: At the age of 40, you will have a life-changing experience. Not a mid-life-crisis-thing, but a God-thing. I won't go into the details because I don't want to ruin it for you. But it will be the most amazing journey of self-discovery. And it will begin with surrendering the ONE THING that DEFINES you—your job, your professional role. I know it sounds ugly, and it will be scary. But you will take this step in faith, and it will be totally worth it!

After nearly 10 years in the Director role, you will start to question if this is what you want. It will seem to be what people want FOR you. In fact, some people will try to convince you that you should pursue the next step in the career ladder. Well-intentioned people will try to convince you that this is what you want as well. But it won't be, and there will be no denying it. You will struggle with the conflict between your heart, mind, and ears, but you will ultimately follow your heart, receive confirmation, and decide to step down from the Director role. It will be your best decision ever!

Note to Self: Once you find that place where your passion and purpose collide, there will be no denying that THAT is the place you are intended to serve. Once you find your lane, stay in it! *Trust me.* You will veer left and veer right a little along the way, but the veering will be just enough to remind you where your lane is. Keep your feet on the path that has been marked for you.

Because of your experience and relationships within the organization, you will be called to serve in various capacities. You will have the opportunity to serve as Interim Director and lead the team through some pretty significant transitions. It will be natural to put your old Director-mask back on, but don't do it! That is not what the team will need from you. They will simply need you to be the person they can trust to lead them through the transition. You will achieve this by creating an interim strategic plan, committing to regular communication and transparency, and being yourself. You will also find that the more you acknowledge your own weaknesses and failures, the more people will trust you. You will learn that people are more comfortable being themselves when you are yourself and not trying to be perfect. This seems to give them permission to share their hopes, dreams, and fears, and opens the door to forming authentic relationships.

Final Note to Self: Twenty-two years into your career and marriage, you will discover the Enneagram which will serve as an incredibly powerful tool to help you learn more about yourself, navigate your relationships, and understand the real work that lies ahead of you. For the last decade, you have known and described yourself as a *reflector*. You value the time and ability to reflect on situations, and this "space" is where you do your best thinking (and planning). But the Enneagram has helped you realize that you are not just an introvert who needs to be away from people and busyness to think, reflect, and rejuvenate; you genuinely crave stillness, and it is essential to quiet your mind, to provide clarity so you can connect and engage in the most fruitful way. You will discover that intentional pauses allow you to see and experience things you wouldn't otherwise. They are critical to reminding you to focus less on what you do and more of who YOU really are. This, my dear, is where you will find the greatest freedom and wholeness, in being your True Self. To quote Ralph Waldo Emerson, "To be yourself in a world that is constantly trying to make you something else is the greatest accomplishment."

Enjoy the journey!

Beth